T0233701

Vestibular Migraine

Stephen Wetmore • Allan Rubin

Editors

Vestibular Migraine

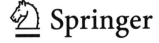 Springer

Editors
Stephen Wetmore, MD, MBA
Otolaryngology
West Virginia University School
of Medicine
Morgantown, WV
USA

Allan Rubin, MD, PhD
Northwest Ohio ENT Consultants
Perrysburg, OH
USA

ISBN 978-3-319-35744-7   ISBN 978-3-319-14550-1   (eBook)
DOI 10.1007/978-3-319-14550-1
Springer Cham Heidelberg New York Dordrecht London

Printed on acid-free paper

Springer is part of Springer Science+Business Media (www.springer.com)

Preface

Vestibular migraine is a term that only in the past several years has become accepted as a clinical diagnosis. Nevertheless, this particular disease classification and the associated diagnostic criteria are still approached with skepticism by some in the medical community.

The idea of dizziness being associated with migraine was mentioned over 50 years ago. It was then thought to be strictly part of basilar migraine headaches. It is now appreciated that this association of dizziness as part of a migraine aura represents only a small percentage of patients with vestibular migraine. It is believed by many clinicians dealing with dizziness that vestibular migraine may be the third most common cause of dizziness after benign paroxysmal positional vertigo and vestibular neuronitis. Furthermore, vestibular migraine has a variety of presentations and can present with other causes of dizziness, such as post-concussive dizziness.

Although a diagnosis of vestibular migraine has been accepted in the field of otolaryngology, there still remains a great deal of skepticism among some neurologists. This is primarily due to the usage of the term migraine as defined by the International Classification of Headache Disorders. Recently physicians representing the Barany Society and International Headache Society have published guidelines to define both definite vestibular migraine as well as probable vestibular migraine. In addition, the most recent edition of the International Classification has published the definite vestibular migraine guidelines in its appendix as a prelude to official acceptance of this entity.

The purpose of this book is to provide the physician with information that can be used to determine whether the patient's vestibular symptoms can be explained as part of the migraine phenomenon. The first chapter will provide the practitioner with information about making a diagnosis of migraine headaches and will include material needed to understand the complex condition known as migraine. The next chapter will provide the practitioner with current ideas of how to make the diagnosis of vestibular migraine. The following chapter provides historic information about how the phenomenon of vestibular migraine was developed along with theories on the pathophysiologic phenomena that cause dizziness in migraineurs. Vestibular manifestations of migraine in children are discussed in a separate chapter. Treatment options for vestibular migraine will be discussed next. The final chapter will discuss the relationships between vestibular migraine and Meniere's disease.

The authors of this book who come from a multidisciplinary background will provide a comprehensive review of the various aspects of vestibular migraine. Our goal is to provide the reader with sufficient information to consider vestibular migraine in the differential diagnosis of the dizzy patient.

Morgantown, WV, USA   Stephen J. Wetmore, MD, MBA
Perrysburg, OH, USA   Allan Rubin, MD, PhD

Contents

Contributors

Yuri Agrawal, MD Department of Otolaryngology-Head and Neck Surgery, Johns Hopkins, Baltimore, MD, USA

Carey D. Balaban, PhD Departments of Otolaryngology, Neurobiology, Communication Science & Disorders, and Bioengineering, University of Pittsburgh, Pittsburgh, PA, USA

Matthew L. Carlson, MD Department of Otolaryngology Head and Neck Surgery, Mayo Clinic, Rochester, MN, USA

Adam M. Cassis, MD Department of Otolaryngology, West Virginia University Hospital, Morgantown, WV, USA

Sharon L. Cushing, MD, MSc FRCSC Department of Otolaryngology Head and Neck Surgery, The Hospital for Sick Children, University of Toronto, Toronto, ON, Canada

Archie's Cochlear Implant Laboratory, The Hospital for Sick Children, Toronto, ON, Canada

Joseph M. Furman, MD, PhD Departments of Otolaryngology, Neurology, Bioengineering and Physical Theraphy, University of Pittsburgh, Pittsburgh, PA, USA

Hongyan Li, MD, PhD Department of Neurology, University of Toledo College of Medicine and Life Sciences, Toledo, OH, USA

Brian A. Neff, MD Department of Otolaryngology Head and Neck Surgery, Mayo Clinic, Rochester, MN, USA

Allan M. Rubin, MD, PhD Department of Surgery, University of Toledo, Perrysburg, OH, USA

David B. Watson, MD Department of Neurology, WVU Headache Center, West Virginia University School of Medicine, Morgantown, WV, USA

Stephen J. Wetmore, MD, MBA Department of Otolaryngology, West Virginia University Hospital, Morgantown, WV, USA

Migraine Headache

1

David B. Watson

1.1 Epidemiology

Migraine has been repeatedly shown to affect roughly 12 % of the population in the United States with a 3:1 preference toward women [1]. As many as 25 % of women in their mid-20s to mid-40s suffer from migraine attacks. While a family history of migraine is often noted, most migraine disorders do not follow clearly defined Mendelian inheritance patterns. There is an increased risk of migraine in first-degree relatives of 1.5–4 times [2]. Several genes have been identified for relatively rare forms of migraine, in particular the familial hemiplegic migraine (FHM). There are three FHM genes identified, including FHM1, the CACNA1A gene on chromosome 19; FHM2, the ATP1A2 gene on chromosome 1; and FHM3, the SCN1A gene on chromosome 2 [2].

Migraine has been associated with a number of other conditions, including mood and anxiety disorders, epilepsy, stroke, irritable bowel syndrome, and fibromyalgia [3]. Migraine is more prevalent in patients who are Caucasian and those with lower household income [4].

According to the Global Burden of Disease Survey from the World Health Organization [5], migraine is the second leading neurologic cause of disability worldwide as measured by disability-adjusted life years (DALYs) and the leading neurologic cause of DALYs in women. It is the ninth all-condition cause of years lost to disability (YLDs), responsible for over 18 million YLDs. In the United States, the estimated societal costs range from $13 to $31 billion, including direct expenses such as medication, provider visits, emergency room visits, and imaging studies, as well as indirect costs of lost or limited productivity. It is the fifth leading cause for emergency department visits with over four million visits yearly in the United States [6].

1.2 Migraine Phases and Physiology

Although the headache component is often the most obvious and troubling symptom of migraine attacks, four phases of migraine have been described: premonitory phase, aura, migraine, and postdrome. Not all sufferers of migraine will experience all four phases, but it is important to be aware of them as each phase can be of concern to patients and can have significant impact on quality of life. While it is common to think of the phases as occurring in a sequential manner, it is likely that these events share underlying mechanisms and timing.

D.B. Watson, MD
Department of Neurology,
West Virginia University School of Medicine,
Box 9180, Morgantown, WV, 26506, USA
e-mail: dwatson@hsc.wvu.edu

S. Wetmore, A. Rubin (eds.), *Vestibular Migraine*,
DOI 10.1007/978-3-319-14550-1_1, © Springer International Publishing Switzerland 2015

1.2.1   Premonitory Phase

Many patients with migraine will develop symptoms many hours prior to the onset of pain. These symptoms are often consistent between attacks and allow for predictability of the headache onset and may in the future provide targets for new therapies. Common premonitory symptoms include fatigue, mood changes, nausea, neck stiffness, irritability, concentration difficulty, yawning, and phonophobia. These symptoms have been reported in over 80 % of adults.

A variety of hypotheses have been put forward to explain the presence of these symptoms including involvement of the dopaminergic systems and dopamine release and increased hypothalamic activity. Dopamine's role in the premonitory phase is supported by the recognition that many of the side effects of dopamine agonists are similar to common early migraine symptoms, especially nausea, yawning, and drowsiness, and dopamine antagonists such as metoclopramide can be effective treatments for some patients. Hypothalamic involvement is suggested by such symptoms as changes in mood, energy, and appetite. Imaging studies revealed increased blood flow in the region during attacks [7].

1.2.2   Aura

The aura phase of migraine has been the subject of much recent study. The traditional view of aura has been that of symptoms directly preceding the onset of headache pain, but recent evidence has suggested a more cohesive nature of aura to the headache phase with similar or concurrent mechanisms rather than the headache being a direct effect of the presence of the aura.

Various imaging modalities, including SPECT, PET, CT, and MRI, have demonstrated alterations in cerebral blood flow or brain metabolism. Making conclusions challenging, both hypoperfusion and hyperperfusion during aura have been demonstrated, and it is recognized that a vast majority of imaging studies done during aura as part of clinical evaluations show no abnormalities [7].

1.2.3   Headache Phase

As stated above, the headache phase may coincide with the aura phase or occur directly following it. It is the portion of the migraine attack most easily recognizable and where most therapeutic efforts have been aimed. The nature of the headache itself will be described in more detail later in this chapter.

Despite the insensate nature of the brain itself, there are many cranial structures capable of pain sensation. The dura, dural vessels, extracranial vessels, cerebral arteries and venous sinuses, cranial nerves, skin, muscles, and other structures can transmit pain signals. Peripheral pain signals from unmyelinated C fibers travel via the trigeminal nerve to the pons and into the trigeminal nucleus caudalis (TNC). This includes not only signals from dural and meningeal vessels but also from upper cervical roots. The TNC connects centrally to the thalamus with collateral connections to autonomic brainstem nuclei and the hypothalamus. There are also connections from the TNC to the superior salivatory nucleus, which projects to the nasal sinuses and eyes. The wide variety of connections to and from the TNC creates multiple options for referred pain and other symptoms, such as nasal congestion and neck pain during migraine attacks.

The exact triggering mechanism for migraine pain remains unclear. Cortical spreading depression (CSD) occurs when a wave of depolarization moves across the cerebral cortex causing the release of nitric oxide, arachidonic acid, protons, and potassium extracellularly. While CSDs are likely implicated in migraine with aura, their involvement in migraine without aura is less clear. Whether caused by CSDs or other mechanisms, meningeal nociceptors become activated and trigeminal nerve terminals at the dural vessels release various substances, including calcitonin gene-related peptide, substance P, and neurokinin A. Vessel dilatation and inflammation follow, known as sterile neurogenic inflammation, and the trigeminal neurons become activated (peripheral sensitization). These signals are transmitted centrally and patients may experience pain. As pain signaling continues, the second- and third-order neurons may become activated (central sensitization). Central sensitization manifests as cutaneous allodynia, or the experience of pain from non-painful stimuli, and patients can report scalp tenderness or even extremity pain. This can be described by patients as difficulty brushing or combing hair, pain with laying the head on a particular side, or neck pain [8]. Burstein and colleagues have demonstrated reduced pain thresholds to mechanical and thermal stimulation and increased thalamic responses to these stimuli during migraine attacks when compared to between attacks [7, 9]. It is possible that these symptoms can confuse the diagnosis of migraine, leading the clinician and patient to describe the headaches as being tension headache. The recognition of migraine early, during the peripheral sensitization phase, and treating prior to the development of central sensitization can lead to better pain abatement, and many antimigraine therapies have been shown to be more effective at addressing the peripheral component of the disorder than central mechanisms [9].

1.2.4 Postdrome Phase

Even after the pain of migraine has resolved, symptoms can persist for hours to days and remain problematic for patients. Commonly reported symptoms include fatigue, weakness, mental sluggishness, and mood alterations. These can be misinterpreted by patients as being side effects of abortive medications and lead to unnecessary abandonment of otherwise appropriate treatments. Both residual hyperperfusion and hypoperfusion have been demonstrated, as well as continued hypothalamic, pontine, and midbrain activation following resolution of migraine pain [7].

1.3 Migraine Diagnoses

The International Classification of Headache Disorders III-Beta [10] has described six main categories of migraine, some with multiple subtypes, including migraine without aura, migraine with aura, chronic migraine, complications of migraine, probable migraine, and episodic syndromes that may be associated with migraine. In addition, there are many proposed migraine subtypes included in the appendix of ICHD-3Beta.

1.3.1 Migraine Without Aura

Migraine without aura (previously called common migraine) is the most common migraine manifestation. Criteria include the following: at least five attacks lasting 4–72 h, with at least two of the following characteristics – unilateral, pulsating, moderate to severe pain, and aggravation by routine physical activity – and at least one of the following, nausea, vomiting, and photophonophobia [10].

1.3.2 Migraine with Aura

Migraine with aura (classical migraine) shares headache features with migraine without aura but includes recurrent, fully reversible attacks of neurologic symptoms, including visual, sensory, or other central nervous system symptoms. Typical aura presents as a gradual progression of visual, sensory, or speech symptoms that can last from 5 to 60 min. Different symptoms can occur in succession, and the aura is generally accompanied by, or followed by, a headache within 60 min. Visual disturbance is the most common aura symptom, followed by paresthesias.

1.3.3 Aura Without Headache

Auras can occur independent of headaches as well. Although auras are considered to be part of the migraine spectrum, further evaluation may be warranted to exclude another underlying disorder.

1.3.4 Hemiplegic Migraine

Hemiplegic migraine is a subtype of migraine with aura that includes motor weakness. Motor symptoms can last up to 72 h but must be fully reversible. Other typical aura symptoms may occur as well. Familial forms of hemiplegic migraine have been reported with three causative mutations described. Just as commonly, however, hemiplegic migraine may be a sporadic disorder with no first- or second-degree relatives who are affected [10].

1.3.5 Migraine with Brainstem Aura

Brainstem aura, previously called basilar artery migraine or basilar-type migraine, includes symptoms referable to brainstem dysfunction in addition to typical aura symptoms. Brainstem aura symptoms include dysarthria, vertigo, tinnitus, hypacusis, diplopia, ataxia, or altered consciousness. When these symptoms are present, it is important to exclude secondary causes of brainstem symptoms prior to labeling them as brainstem aura.

1.3.6 Retinal Migraine

Aura symptoms of monocular visual disturbance, such as blindness or scotoma, are referred to as retinal migraine. Care must be taken to ensure that patients are actually experiencing monocular symptoms rather than unilateral visual field symptoms. Again, diagnostic evaluation may be necessary to exclude other causes of transient monocular vision loss.

It is important to remember that each of the above migraine subtypes is not exclusive of one another. Patients may experience migraine without aura as well as migraine with typical aura, hemiplegic migraine, etc. over the course of different attacks.

1.3.7 Chronic Migraine

Migraine is usually an infrequent, episodic disorder. However, it can progress into a more frequent form known as chronic migraine (CM). In general, CM requires the presence of 15 days per month of headache for 3 months, with migraine features present on at least eight of those days. A variety of causes for the progression to CM have been reported, with the most common being the overuse of medication intended to abort migraine attacks. Medication overuse has been described with opiates, benzodiazepines, triptans, ergotamines, butalbital combinations, acetaminophen, and over-the-counter (OTC) combinations. Other factors involved in the development of CM include lower educational status, obesity, diabetes, arthritis, high caffeine intake, snoring, and high baseline headache frequency [11].

A variety of other migraine subtypes have been described with varying levels of epidemiologic evidence. Cyclic vomiting syndrome, abdominal migraine, benign paroxysmal vertigo, and benign paroxysmal torticollis have now been included as official ICHD-3 migraine subtypes. Other subtypes which have been included in the appendix of the classification include pure menstrual migraine without aura, menstrual-related migraine without aura, and episodic syndromes that may be associated with migraine, such as infantile colic and alternating hemiplegia of childhood [10].

1.4 Evaluation of the Migraine Patient

Migraine symptomatology can be severe and dramatic, often convincing patients and providers that an underlying, discoverable mechanism for them must be present. However, migraine remains a clinical- and history-driven diagnosis. Workup for a patient with migraine without aura or migraine with typical aura may include only a detailed medical history and physical exam. According to the American Academy of Neurology Quality Standards [12], only 0.7 % of patients who present with migraine symptoms and have normal exams will have abnormalities on brain imaging. Patients presenting with progressive or changing headache patterns; atypical aura symptoms, such as motor weakness or brainstem symptoms; or aura symptoms that do not resolve within 60 min may warrant further imaging evaluations.

1.5 Treatment

The treatment of migraine is often a multifaceted approach, involving abortive therapies, preventative medications, and behavioral changes. The overall choice of therapy depends on a variety of factors, including headache severity and frequency, patient comorbidities, medication side effect tolerability, and patient preference. Developing an appropriate treatment plan requires a comprehensive evaluation of the patient's headache history, medical history, family and social structure, and insurance coverage.

1.5.1 Abortive Medications

The goals of acute or abortive treatment of migraine headache are to relieve pain and to restore function as quickly as possible. As a general rule, abortive medications are most effective when taken early in the course of the headache, but this should not be misinterpreted to mean that patients should not treat headaches if they were unable to intervene early. It is important to understand the nature and severity of the headaches that the patient is experiencing in order to help determine the nature of the treatment. Patients with mild to moderate migraine headaches may be adequately treated with simple analgesics such as ibuprofen or naproxen, but those whose headaches are typically moderate to severe should be started on a more "aggressive" therapy, such as triptans or ergotamines. Acute treatment can be categorized as nonspecific or migraine-specific therapy.

1.5.1.1 Nonspecific Therapies

Nonsteroidal anti-inflammatories, such as aspirin, ibuprofen, naproxen, and diclofenac, have been shown to be effective options for many patients with migraine. Often, they are used in combination with antiemetics such as metoclopramide or prochlorperazine. If effective for the individual, they can be advantageous as they are generally less expensive than migraine-specific therapy and well tolerated. A powdered version of diclofenac has been shown to be effective for migraine headache. Ketorolac, in an IV formulation, is commonly used in the urgent care and emergency room setting to abort headaches. This drug exhibits a potential risk of gastrointestinal bleeding and cardiovascular risk that may limit its use in some patients.

Dopamine antagonists, such as antiemetics and neuroleptics, may also be effective in providing relief for the headache pain and also nausea. Prochlorperazine is available parenterally, orally, and in suppository formulations, and metoclopramide is available in an oral formulation. These drugs can be used in combination with NSAIDs or triptans if necessary and are generally well tolerated, although akathisia or sedation can occur. Other antiemetics such as ondansetron and promethazine may be helpful in the treatment of nausea associated with migraine but show limited efficacy in headache relief [13].

Combination therapies, such as those available over the counter, typically involve some combination of aspirin, acetaminophen, and caffeine. Although these combinations may be effective for patients with mild to moderate pain, the risk of worsening headache and the development of medication overuse headache is significant, and particular care should be taken to limit their use. Minimal evidence is available to support the use of butalbital-containing medications for migraine despite its widespread use. Butalbital carries significant risk for medication overuse headache, it is sedating, and sudden withdrawal can lead to seizures. Certain European countries have eliminated the availability of butalbital-containing medications, and they are generally not recommended for routine use in headache medicine.

1.5.1.2 Migraine-Specific Therapies

Triptans are selective serotonin 5-hydroxytryptamine 1B and 1D receptor agonists. Their proposed mechanisms of action include inhibition of trigeminal nerve terminal release of inflammatory peptides, intracranial arterial vasoconstriction, and brainstem neuronal inhibition via presynaptic dorsal horn stimulation [13]. Seven unique triptan molecules are available in the United States, and all have proven efficacy for the acute treatment of migraine in randomized clinical trials (RCTs). All seven compounds are available in oral formulations, while some are available intranasally, subcutaneously, and transdermally. The triptans are considered a first-line therapy for moderate to severe migraine headaches, and early intervention is recommended for best results, but the efficacy later in the headache is still sufficient and is still encouraged if necessary. Selection of route of administration can depend on severity of the headache, timing, tolerability, concurrent symptoms, and patient preference. Patients with sudden onset and rapidly escalating pain, or those who awaken with headaches, may especially benefit from intranasal or subcutaneous administration, as well as those with significant nausea limiting the ability to use oral forms. Fear of needles and discomfort from injections may limit the use of subcutaneous forms. Patients with a history of vascular disease, including coronary artery disease, cerebrovascular disease, and peripheral vascular disease, should not use triptans due to their vasoconstrictive effects. Those persons without a previous history of vascular disease but with significant risk factors such as smoking, obesity, or diabetes may warrant appropriate cardiac evaluations prior to administration of triptans (Table 1.1).

Dihydroergotamine remains a widely used ergot in the management of acute migraine pain. It is less receptor specific than the triptans and, therefore, is more prone to side effects such as nausea, but some patients find it to be more efficacious than triptans. It is available in a nasal spray formulation as well as an injectable that can be given subcutaneously, intramuscularly, or intravenously.

For patients with intractable migraine headache who are in an inpatient setting, dihydroergotamine can be given repeatedly over a number of days.

1.5.2 Preventive Medication

When patients suffer with frequent migraine headaches, they may become candidates for the use of preventive medication options. Although there is no absolute number of headache days per month threshold, a general cutoff has traditionally been at two headache days per week. This has

Table 1.1 FDA-approved triptan options for acute treatment of migraine headache

Triptan	Formulations	Dosages (mg)
Sumatriptan	Oral	25, 50, 100, 85 with 500 mg naproxen
	Nasal spray	5, 20
	Subcutaneous injection	4, 6
	Transdermal	6.5
Rizatriptan	Oral	5, 10
	Oral melting tablet	5, 10
Zolmitriptan	Oral	2.5, 5
	Oral melting tablet	2.5, 5
	Nasal spray	2.5, 5
Naratriptan	Oral	1, 2.5
Eletriptan	Oral	20, 40
Almotriptan	Oral	6.25, 12.5
Frovatriptan	Oral	2.5

come under scrutiny recently as there are other variables that factor into the decision, including severity of the headache, associated symptoms, success of acute treatments, and patient preference. Some patients may desire daily preventive medication over even the occasional severe, disabling headache, while others may prefer to treat acutely rather than take daily medicine. Of note, the presence of nine or more headache days per month has been shown to be an independent risk factor for the progression to chronic migraine, so serious consideration for prevention may be warranted in patients with what is commonly referred to as high-frequency episodic migraine.

There are several general principles for the selection and use of preventive medications. Start the medication at a low dose, and then progressively increase the dose over time until headaches are sufficiently limited or side effects are no longer tolerable. Preventives should be maintained for at least 2–3 months before a determination of efficacy is made. Selection of which agent to use can be aided by looking for the "therapeutic two for one," or choosing a medication that can treat both the migraines and another issue for the patient (depression, insomnia, hypertension).

The US Food and Drug Administration has only approved four agents for the prevention of migraine: topiramate, valproic acid, propranolol,

Table 1.2 Preventive medication options for prevention of migraine and level of evidence [12, 13, 18]

Preventive medication	Common dosages (mg)	Level of evidence
Divalproex sodium/sodium valproate[a]	250–1,500	A
Topiramate[a]	50–200	A
Metoprolol	50–150	A
Propranolol[a]	80–240	A
Timolol[a]	20–60	A
Amitriptyline	10–150	B
Venlafaxine	75–225	B
Atenolol	50–200	B
Nadolol	20–160	B
Lisinopril	10–20	C
Candesartan	16	C

Adapted from Silberstein et al. [12]
A = established efficacy (2 or more class 1 trials)
B = probably efficacy (1 class 1 trial or 2 class 2 studies)
C = probably efficacy (1 class 2 study)
[a]FDA approval

and timolol. A number of other medications are commonly used, including other antiepileptics and antihypertensives and antidepressants. Recently the American Academy of Neurology and the American Headache Society published a review of the evidence for preventive medications, which are summarized in Table 1.2.

1.5.2.1 Antiepileptic Drugs (AEDs)
Topiramate
Topiramate was initially approved by the US FDA for the treatment of certain epilepsies but has since gained approval for the prevention of migraine. Common doses are between 100 and 200 mg per day, either once or twice daily. It is recommended to start at a lower dose, often 15 or 25 mg, and slowly titrate the dose to avoid side effects. The most commonly reported side effects are paresthesias, or a pins and needles sensation in the hands, feet, or perioral region, cognitive changes, and appetite suppression or taste changes. Carbonated beverages are often perceived as being flat or having a metallic taste. Topiramate can increase the risk of renal calculus formation and should be used with caution or avoided in those with a history of stones. It has been reported to induce acute angle closure

glaucoma, and reports of severe eye pain should lead to discontinuation of therapy and urgent ophthalmologic evaluation. Like many of the preventives used, it shows roughly a 50 % reduction of headache frequency in 50 % of those treated.

Valproate
Valproate, although FDA approved for migraine prevention, has limited use due to side effects, necessary monitoring, and significant evidence as a cause of neural tube defects in pregnancy. It is sometimes an appropriate choice in patients with comorbid epilepsy or psychiatric disease, or when patients have been refractory to other agents. This drug is associated with elevated liver enzymes and hepatitis; laboratory monitoring is recommended. Common side effects include weight gain, tremor, and hair loss. Recommended doses range from 500 to 1,500 mg per day.

Other AEDs
Gabapentin and zonisamide are other antiepileptics that may be appropriate for use. Zonisamide has many similarities to topiramate and is an option when topiramate is limited by side effects. It does have the advantage of a longer half-life allowing once daily dosing. Gabapentin has limited evidence for efficacy in migraine prevention, but its positive effects on sleep and general tolerability make it a tempting option.

1.5.2.2 Antihypertensives
Beta-adrenergic blockers and calcium channel blockers have commonly been used for prevention, and more recently, candesartan, an angiotensin receptor blocker, has shown benefit.

Beta-Adrenergic Blockers
Although propranolol and timolol carry the FDA approval, many different beta-blockers are commonly used, including atenolol and metoprolol. They can be useful in patients who also have hypertension, although it is unclear if they are the best agents for preventing the long-term consequences of hypertension. They can also be useful in patients with comorbid anxiety, as long as depression is not present, as they can worsen depression. Certain beta-blockers are considered

to be probably safe in pregnancy, and they may be an option for prevention of migraine in this challenging population.

Calcium Channel Blockers

Verapamil is the most often used drug of this class for prevention of migraine. Evidence for the entire class is limited and has led to a less favorable rating by the AAN/AHS quality standards. Like beta-blockers, it may be useful in patients with hypertension. Common doses range from 80 to 480 mg per day, but side effects of lightheadedness, constipation, and lower-extremity edema can be problematic, and electrocardiogram monitoring with dosage increases is recommended due to the risk of heart block.

1.5.2.3 Antidepressants

Tricyclic antidepressants (TCAs) and serotonin-norepinephrine reuptake inhibitors (SNRIs), more so than SSRIs, have good evidence for the prevention of migraine despite not receiving FDA approval. Amitriptyline is by far the best studied of the TCAs and has consistently shown benefit as a preventive agent. Doses typically range anywhere from 10 to 75 mg but can go up to 150 mg if needed and tolerated. Many patients will benefit from doses much lower than those previously used to treat depression. Common side effects are sedation (which can be used to treat those with significant insomnia) and dry mouth. At typical migraine preventive doses, weight gain is possible but much less likely than at antidepressant ranges. A variety of other TCAs have been used, and some have been suggested to be better tolerated than amitriptyline if side effects are the limiting factor.

Venlafaxine is an SNRI with some evidence to support its use in migraine prevention. Typical doses range from 75 to 225 mg, but it should be started lower and titrated upward to avoid or limit nausea. It may be a very good option for patients with comorbid depression or anxiety. One challenge with the use of venlafaxine is significant vertigo triggered by the discontinuation of the drug. Patients should be cautioned not to stop it abruptly, but dizziness can be seen even with a slow taper [13].

1.5.2.4 Botulinum Toxin for Chronic Migraine

OnabotulinumtoxinA has been extensively studied for the prevention of migraine. It is currently approved for the treatment of chronic migraine (15 days per month or more of headache with 8 days of migraine). Its efficacy has been tested repeatedly in a variety of doses, injection sites, and patient types with varying levels of success. Two large, blinded, and placebo-controlled trials with subjects with chronic migraine showed a significant reduction in headache days and headache hours when compared to placebo when using a "fixed site, fixed dose" approach of 155 units of toxin delivered via 31 specific injection sites covering a number of muscles including the frontalis, temporalis, and trapezius. Potential advantages to patients with chronic migraine include limited systemic side effects and prolonged benefit between treatments. However, costs and insurance coverage limitations, pain, and limited access to qualified injectors may limit its utility [14].

1.5.2.5 Non-pharmacologic and Alternative Options

Not all patients with frequent migraine wish to take prescription preventive medications. A number of non-pharmacologic or alternative therapies have been proven to be effective in reducing the frequency and/or severity of migraine headaches. Biofeedback [15] and cognitive behavioral therapy (CBT) [16] trials have shown benefit for the reduction of migraine headaches, while other promising options include relaxation therapy, physical therapy, massage therapy, and acupuncture [17]. The potential advantage to these approaches is limited risks and side effects as well as potentially returning a level of control back to the patient. However, both biofeedback and CBT require a significant time commitment and dedication to the process, and costs can often create a problem as insurance coverage is often lacking or limited.

While there are many supplements available that are claimed to be helpful to prevent migraine headaches, a few of these "natural" therapies have been reasonably studied and have shown promise. Magnesium, butterbur (*Petasites hybridus* root), coenzyme Q10, riboflavin, and feverfew have evidence to support their use in the prevention of migraine headaches. Magnesium has had mixed results in a variety of trials, which may be related to differing salt forms (citrate, aspartate) and dosing. It is inexpensive and generally well tolerated, although diarrhea can be a limiting side effect. Butterbur root has promising data to support its effectiveness and is well tolerated. There are, however, safety concerns due to the presence of pyrrolizidine alkaloids in the *Petasites* plant that can be hepatotoxic [18].

Conclusion

Migraine, with its high prevalence, noted disability, and significant costs, is an important disorder not only to those who suffer but also to society as a whole. The complex yet incompletely understood pathophysiology of migraine leads to a disorder with varying symptomatology, including headache, environmental sensitivities, motion intolerance, gastrointestinal difficulties, mood alterations, as well as many other manifestations. While headache is often the most recognizable symptom, the underlying mechanisms of the disease can lead to a wide array of neurologic signs and symptoms, including vertigo, which will be described in detail in the remainder of this text. An ability to properly diagnose migraine can improve the chances for the patient to obtain significant reduction in pain and disability. Treatment options include pharmaceutical preventives and abortives, natural therapies, and physical and behavioral therapies. As the understanding of migraine mechanisms improve, the hope for patients and providers is that the options for treatment improve as well.

References

1. Lipton RB, Bigal ME, Diamond M, Freitag F, Reed ML, Stewart WF, on behalf of the AMPP Advisory Group. Migraine prevalence, disease burden, and the need for preventive therapy. Neurology. 2007;68:343–9.
2. Ferrari MD, Dichgans M. Genetics of primary headaches. In: Silberstein SD, Lipton RB, Dodick DW, editors. Wolff's headache and other head pain. 8th ed. New York: Oxford University Press; 2008.
3. Lipton RB, Scher AI, Silberstein SD, Bigal ME. Migraine diagnosis and comorbidity. In: Silberstein SD, Lipton RB, Dodick DW, editors. Wolff's headache and other head pain. 8th ed. New York: Oxford University Press; 2008.
4. Lipton RB, Bigal ME, Diamond M, Freitag F, Reed ML, Stewart WF, on behalf of the AMPP Advisory Group. Migraine prevalence, disease burden, and the need for preventive therapy. Neurology. 2007;68:343–9.
5. Health statistics and information systems – regional estimates for 2000–2011. [internet] 2014. Available from: http://www.who.int/healthinfo/global_burden_disease/estimates_regional/en/index1.html.
6. Smitherman TA, Burch R, Sheikh J, Loder E. The prevalence, impact, and treatment of migraine and severe headaches in the United States: a review of statistics from national surveillance studies. Headache. 2013;53:427–36.
7. Charles A. The evolution of a migraine attack – a review of recent evidence. Headache. 2013;53(2):413–9.
8. Ward TN. Migraine diagnosis and pathophysiology. Contin Lifelong Learn Neurol. 2012;18(4):753–63.
9. Burstein R, Jakubowski M, Garcia-Nicas E, Kainz V, Bajwa Z, Hargreaves R, Becerra L, Borsook D. Thalamic sensitization transforms localized pain into widespread allodynia. Ann Neurol. 2010;68(1):81–91.
10. Headache Classification Committee of the International Headache Society. The international classification of headache disorders, 3rd edition (beta version). Cephalalgia. 2013;33(9):629–808.
11. Tepper S. Medication overuse headache. Contin Lifelong Learn Neurol. 2012;18(4):807–22.
12. Silberstein S, Holland S, Freitag F. Evidence-based guideline update: pharmacologic treatment for episodic migraine prevention in adults: report of the quality standards subcommittee of the American Academy of Neurology and the American Headache Society. Neurology. 2012;78:1337–45.
13. Rizzoli P. Acute and preventive treatment of migraine. Contin Lifelong Learn Neurol. 2012;18(4):764–82.
14. Diener HC, Dodick DW, Aurora SK, Turkel CC, DeGryse RE, Lipton RB, Silberstein SD, Brin MF, PREEMPT 2 Chronic Migraine Study Group. OnabotulinumtoxinA for treatment of chronic migraine: results from the double-blind, randomized, placebo-controlled phase of the PREEMPT 2 trial. Cephalalgia. 2010;30(7):804–14.
15. Nestoriuc Y, Martin A. Efficacy of biofeedback for migraine: a meta-analysis. Pain. 2007;128(1–2):111–27.
16. Campbell JK, Penzien DB, Wall EM. Evidence-based guidelines for migraine headache: behavioral and physical treatments. US Headache Consortium. 2000. http://tools.aan.com/professionals/practice/pdfs/gl0089.pdf. Accessed by Jan 6, 2015.
17. Chopra R, Robert T, Watson D. Non-pharmacologic and pharmacologic prevention of episodic migraine and chronic daily headache. WV Med J. 2012;108(3):90–3.
18. Silberstein SD, Freitag FG, Bigal ME. Migraine treatment. In: Silberstein SD, Lipton RB, Dodick DW, editors. Wolff's headache and other head pain. 8th ed. New York: Oxford University Press; 2008.

Hongyan Li

2.1 Introduction

Vestibular migraine has been well recognized as a common episodic vertiginous disorder [1–3]. Until recently, clinicians have been often challenged by a lack of unequivocal and generally accepted criteria to define this entity. Uncertainty with the diagnosis and inconsistency among the caring physicians, mainly neurologists and otolaryngologists, are common. These difficulties in clinical practice are at least partially attributed to the continuing limitations in understanding the mechanisms of this common disorder. Even the fundamental pathophysiological mechanisms of migraine are still yet to be completely revealed [4, 5].

It is important to mention that the clinical and scientific interests about *migraine* have extended far beyond its original meaning of *unilateral headache* (or *hemikrania* in Greek) [6]. Currently, migraine often refers to clinical conditions or disorders that are characterized by a combination of several featured symptoms. These include headaches, intolerance to some sensory inputs, and the subsequently developed reactions to these discomforts. *Vestibular symptoms and signs,* such as vertigo, dizziness, unsteadiness, and nystagmus, are among the most consistent and significant presentations during typical migraine attacks in many patients [1, 2, 7]. Meanwhile, prominent vestibular symptoms can also be related to a few special neurological disorders that, as to be discussed later in this chapter, demonstrate significant overlap with migraine in their clinical presentations. Furthermore, these symptoms can be the manifestation of a coexisting disorder besides migraine and become unmasked during migraine attacks. To diagnose vestibular migraine, clinicians must be able to recognize and differentiate these entities from each other. As part of the progress toward better understanding of vestibular migraine, a diagnostic guideline for vestibular migraine has been published and is to be included in the soon-to-be-published third version of International Classification of Headache Disorders (ICHD-III) [8].

This chapter will focus on the clinical reasoning process toward diagnosing vestibular migraine and its related conditions. Clinical implications of the recently available diagnostic criteria will be discussed.

2.2 The Definition of Vestibular Migraine

The *vestibular system* deals with spatial orientation and the motion status of the head. Its functions are critical for the stabilizations of gaze,

H. Li, MD, PhD
Department of Neurology, University of Toledo
College of Medicine and Life Sciences,
MS1195, 3000 Arlington Avenue,
Toledo, OH 43614, USA
e-mail: hongyan.li@utoledo.edu

and head and body postures, in both static and dynamic conditions. Through its peripheral and central components and connections, this system allows subjects to perceive and to react to the changes of head position and motion status. This ensures gaze fixation at the interested target and body balance allowing the subject to execute the proposed voluntary activities. Vestibular dysfunctions, which may be secondary to an interruption at a peripheral or central location of the vestibular system, lead to intense discomforts [9]. These discomforts are secondary to impaired perception of head orientation and motion. This leads to an inability to maintain or change body balance, inability to maintain gaze fixation, and the subsequent alteration of cognition and autonomic reactions.

There are many descriptions about *vestibular symptoms and signs*. These symptoms and signs have to be weighed carefully in order to determine their vestibular relevance [10]. While vertigo, unsteadiness, and nystagmus are more indicative of vestibular origins, symptoms like fainting, lightheadedness, and wooziness are more suggestive of non-vestibular causes. *Vertigo* is an illusory perception of spatial orientation and head motion that occurs when the subject's cognitive prediction does not match with the actual sensory inputs [11]. It can be related to a variety of causes or mechanisms and has different types. Some objective signs, such as nystagmus and directional falls, more likely indicate a vestibular-related dysfunction. Physical findings, such as heat tilt, can be secondary to many underlying reasons. In addition, patients may also suffer from significant autonomic and psychiatric complications as reactions to vestibular dysfunction. Examples of such complications are nausea, vomiting, diaphoresis, phobia and intolerance to head motion, anticipating anxiety, and depression. International efforts toward a standardized documentation of vestibular disorders have resulted in a semiological classification of vestibular symptoms [10]. This classification was proposed by the Bárány Society and is to be adopted in clinical practice. It includes definitions of a variety of vestibular symptoms and recommendations for standardized documentation of patients' vestibular complaints.

Although the mechanisms of migraine remain poorly understood, the current general consensus is that migraine is fundamentally a neural phenomenon and represents an overly sensitized, hyperactive, and dysfunctional status of the central nervous system [3, 5, 12]. During migraine attacks, the brain becomes unusually sensitive and is inappropriately reactive such that even normal levels of sensory input become intolerable.

Vestibular migraine is a type of migraine disorder that is characterized by prominent vestibular symptoms during a typical attack. The association of migraine and vertigo has been well recognized for many years [1, 2, 7, 13–17]. It has been estimated that vertigo is three to four times more common in migraine sufferers than in controls [1]. About 30–50 % of migraine patients also have dizziness [1, 3]. Intolerance to the motion of head and eyes is frequently reported by migraine patients. Those vestibular symptoms are in fact the cardinal presentations of migraine and are equivalent to the other typical migraine symptoms. The migraine-related vestibular symptoms should not be simply regarded as *migraine aura* [8] since those symptoms barely occur prior to the onset of headache. Instead, they are usually prominent throughout the entire courses of migraine attacks. Although most migraine patients have both headaches and dizziness, many may suffer more from vestibular discomforts than from headaches and some may even have no headache but dizziness and other migraine-related symptoms.

2.3 The Diagnostic Criteria for Migraine and Vestibular Migraine

Although vestibular migraine has been recognized for many years and has been considered as one of the most common causes of vestibular symptoms, it has yet to be adopted as an independent diagnosis. It is not listed in the currently used second edition of International Classification of Headache Disorders (ICHD-II) [18]. The ICHD-II does include a few migraine conditions that may present with prominent vestibular symptoms, such as *basilar-type migraine* and *benign paroxysmal vertigo of childhood*. Vestibular symptoms can be also associated with *headaches attributed to Chiari malformation type 1, disorders of ears/eyes,* and *panic disorders*. Vestibular symptoms may also present with *familial hemiplegic migraine* and *episodic ataxia type 2*. Migraine patients who have prominent vestibular symptoms may be sometimes ambiguously diagnosed with *migraine variant*.

2.3.1 The Diagnostic Criteria for Migraine

Migraine has been classified as a primary type of headache in the ICHD-II [18]. Migraine includes two major subtypes – *migraine with aura* and *migraine without aura*. The *typical migraine headache* has at least two of the following features: (1) unilateral location, (2) pulsating quality, (3) moderate to severe intensity, and (4) aggravation by or resulting in avoidance of routine physical activities. The *typical symptoms associated with migraine headaches* are (1) nausea and/or vomiting and (2) hypersensitivities to sound (phonophobia) and/or light (photophobia). *Migraine aura* is defined as a complex of recurrent and fully reversible focal neurological symptoms (positive or negative) that develop gradually in 5–20 min prior to or at the onset of migraine headaches and last for less than 60 min. The most commonly reported migraine auras are transient interruptions of vision, altered sensation in face or body, and disturbance of speech.

According to the ICHD-II [18], the diagnosis of *migraine without aura* can be made with a patient whose headaches have fulfilled the following criteria: (1) at least 5 typical headache attacks that demonstrate at least 2 of the 4 aforementioned features and last for 4–72 h, (2) at least 1 of the typical symptoms associated with migraine headaches, and (3) no alternative cause. A diagnosis of *migraine with aura* can be made if a patient presents with at least 2 typical migraine headaches with typical migraine aura(s) that cannot be attributed to another disorder. Migraine has many variants that can be identified using the ICHD-II diagnostic criteria as reference.

In clinical practice, migraine may present with nonspecific and equivocal features. For example, the location of the headache at onset can be exclusively on one side, alternating unilateral, or bilateral. The distribution of headache may change during one migraine attack or through many attacks over time and so does the lateralization. The headaches may be described as sharp, stabbing, or piercing instead of throbbing or pounding. Besides photophobia and phonophobia, the migraine patients are often also unable to tolerate strong odor, head motion, and the visualization of moving objects. Severe nausea often leads to vomiting and inadequate intake of food and liquid, which may eventually cause dehydration, hypotension, and electrolyte disturbances. Migraine patients with chronic and refractory attacks may develop depression, anxiety, and other psychiatric or psychological symptoms [19–23]. These symptoms may eventually become so debilitating and overwhelming that they replace headache and other cardinal features as the most prominent comorbidity.

2.3.2 The Diagnostic Criteria for Vestibular Migraine

Vestibular symptoms, such as vertigo and unsteadiness, are common during migraine attacks and may persist between attacks. Patients with migraine may develop dizziness or vertigo, such as feeling self-rotation or rotation of the surroundings. In some patients nystagmus may be witnessed. Instead of using the word "vertigo," many patients describe their dizziness as unsteadiness, wooziness, wobbling, imbalance, drunken, or merely moving sensation. Migraine-associated dizziness can be positional or non-positional. Migraine patients are typically unable to tolerate head motion that exacerbates their dizziness, headaches, and nausea. The orientation to their head positions and surroundings is also felt differently. Those symptoms indicate that the interrupted perception of space and head motion is likely behind the dysfunctional vestibular system. This may be at least partially responsible for the complaints of feeling cloudy-minded, having difficulty concentrating, being confused, and suffering from transient global amnesia.

In 2009, the Committee for the Classification of Vestibular Disorders of the Bárány Society published a consensus classification of vestibular symptoms as the initial effort toward the first edition of International Classification of Vestibular Disorders (ICVD-I) [10]. According to this consensus, *vestibular symptoms can be classified into vertigo, dizziness, vestibulo-visual symptoms, and postural symptoms. Vertigo, or internal vertigo*, is an illusory sensation of self-motion or a sensation of distorted self-motion during head stationary or normal movement statuses. *Dizziness* is defined as a distorted or impaired perception of spatial orientation without sensation of motion. Both vertigo and dizziness are further subclassified on the basis of whether the occurrence is *spontaneous* or is *triggered* by head position, visual stimulation, sound, glottis/nose-pinched Valsalva maneuver, arising orthostasis, and other conditions. *Vestibulo-visual symptoms* are the visual distortions caused by an impaired vestibular system or its interaction with the visual system. Symptoms under this category include external vertigo, oscillopsia, visual lag, visual tilt, and movement-induced blurriness. *Postural symptoms* include unsteadiness, directional pulsion, and balance-related fall and near fall.

More recently, further international efforts have resulted in another consensus about diagnosing vestibular migraine [8]. The consensus includes diagnostic criteria that were jointly prepared by the Committee for Classification of Vestibular Disorders of the Bárány Society and the Migraine Classification Subcommittee of the International Headache Society. Vestibular migraine will be adopted as a new disorder in ICHD-III that is expected to be released in 2014.

According to the purposed *diagnostic criteria for vestibular migraine* [8], the diagnosis of vestibular migraine is based on the presence of the following conditions: (1) recurrent vestibular symptoms, (2) a current or previous history of migraine, (3) a temporal correlation between those vestibular symptoms and migraine attacks, and (4) exclusion of another cause of the vestibular symptoms. The diagnosis of *vestibular*

migraine can be made when all of the following requirements are fulfilled.

2.3.3 Requirements for Diagnosing Vestibular Migraine [8]

A. *Vestibular symptoms:* (1) at least 5 episodes, (2) moderate or severe intensity, and (3) duration of 5 min to 72 h.
B. *Migraine history:* (1) current or previous; (2) fulfill the ICHD-II criteria for migraine with or without aura.
C. *Migraine features:* a demonstration of at least 1 of the following characteristics during at least 50 % of the vestibular episodes: (1) headache with at least 2 of the following features – unilateral location, pulsating quality, moderate or severe pain intensity, and aggravation by routine physical activities – (2) photophobia and phonophobia; and (3) visual aura.
D. *Not better accounted for by another vestibular or ICHD diagnosis:* There is no other disorder that may account for the vestibular symptoms better than migraine.

In addition to vestibular migraine, the Bárány Society has also proposed a diagnosis of *possible vestibular migraine* when only three of the above four requirements, i.e., *A, B, and D or A, C, and D*, are fulfilled [8].

2.4 Clinical Approaches to Diagnosing Vestibular Migraine

The diagnosis of a neurological disorder involves a well-organized reasoning process composed of a series of systemic approaches. It begins with obtaining a detailed history relevant to the presented neurological symptoms. A comprehensive physical examination, including general, neurological, and neuro-otological evaluations [24], is carefully performed when the history is taken. When neurological deficits are identified, the history taking and physical examination should be extended in order to localize the corresponding

Fig. 2.1 Algorithm
of approaching diagnosis
of vestibular migraine [8]

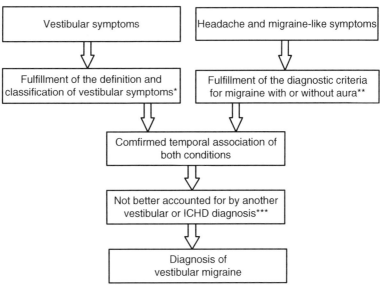

*   Bisdorff et al. [10]
**   International headache society classification subcommittee. [18]
*** Lempert et al. [8]

lesion to the deficits. Once the localization has been completed, efforts are made to identify the underlying cause of the lesion. Then, based on a comprehensive understanding of all the significant clinical findings, a likely diagnosis is proposed together with a list of differential diagnoses. References to the accepted criteria are made in the next step to determine if the clinical findings would fulfill the known standards for diagnosing the proposed disorder. When necessary, supplementary studies, such as radiological, physiological, biochemical, and surgical investigations, may be selected to facilitate diagnosis and to exclude alternative diagnoses. The following algorithm is prepared to assist the clinical approach toward diagnosing vestibular migraine (Fig. 2.1).

2.4.1   Recognition and Confirmation of Vestibular Symptoms

When a patient presents with dizziness or other apparent vestibular symptoms, one should first determine if these symptoms are indeed vestibular related [25]. The answers are often found in reviewing the patient's history that needs to be comprehensive and detailed. The presenting

symptoms are questioned from all possible aspects in order to understand their possible vestibular relevance and values in localization and diagnosis. For example, a vestibular relevance is strongly suggested when the symptoms include directional spinning and a sensation of self-motion or unsteadiness with directional pulsion. In contrast, the vestibular relevance is likely poor if the dizziness is reported as feeling lightheaded and fainting.

When the vestibular symptoms have been verified in reference to the recommended definitions and classifications [10], the patient should be further questioned regarding a few other symptoms that are frequently associated with vestibular disorders, such as gait disturbance, visual disturbance, nausea, tinnitus, hearing loss, earache, etc. These symptoms can be important for the differential diagnosis. Questions should cover the entire course of progression for each symptom starting from its onset.

Once the presenting vestibular symptoms and their related conditions are understood, the possibly involved neural structures need to be localized and a list of possible diagnoses formulated. For example, recurrent episodic vertigo, which is characterized as brief intense spinning attacks and only associated with head turning toward a certain side in supine position, is indicative of positional irritation of the ipsilateral posterior semicircular canal and is most likely related to canalithiasis or cupulolithiasis, i.e., benign paroxysmal positional vertigo. The concurrence of recurrent episodic spinning-type vertigo and unsteadiness with directional pulsion and ipsilateral ear fullness, loud tinnitus, and hearing loss suggests the involvement of ipsilateral peripheral vestibular and auditory components. In this case, Menière's disease or acoustic neuroma should be considered. Meanwhile, the migraine-related vestibular symptoms are often poorly localized or grossly localized to the brainstem or cerebellum. As a matter of fact, when a relevant focal lesion is clearly indicated, migraine will unlikely be the diagnosis. However, migraine should be highly suspected when the dizziness is correlated with episodic headache attacks, sensitivity to light and/or noise, nausea, and poor tolerance to head motion. Such a possibility needs to be also considered when episodic headaches and other migraine-like symptoms are identified even when these symptoms may not coincide with the current dizziness.

2.4.2 Recognition and Confirmation of Migraine History

When the vestibular systems are confirmed, the patient should be asked for a possible previous or current history of headaches. If such a history does exist, detailed headache features should be inquired by means of the same approaches toward vestibular symptoms as previously discussed. Efforts are also made to explore headache-associated symptoms, such as visual aura, nausea, photophobia, and phonophobia. If these symptoms fulfill the ICHD-II criteria for diagnosing migraine with or without aura and alternative diagnosis can be excluded, the existence of migraine is recognized [18]. All the patients with migraine headache should be asked for any vestibular symptoms and those symptoms, if present, should be further assessed for their vestibular relevance with the previously discussed criteria.

Since sometimes a history of migraine can be difficult to clearly diagnose, a systemic approach following the clinician's persistent efforts to identify and localize neurological symptoms and to formulate and refine the diagnostic hypothesis is again the key for uncovering the critical elements for migraine diagnosis.

2.4.3 Correlation Between Vestibular Symptoms and Migraine

After recognizing the coexistence of both vestibular symptoms and a history of migraine, the clinician should attempt to find out whether this coexistence is related to the same underlying etiology or is merely a coincidence. The diagnosis of vestibular migraine requires the recognition of a temporal correlation between vestibular symptoms and migraine [8]. Once again, a careful review of all the relevant information from the entire history and physiological examination is essential to determine the relationship between these clinical symptoms. For example, a migraine patient may also suffer from vertigo related to a compressive meningioma at the cerebellopontine angle region on one side. In a case like this, both headache and vertigo can happen together at times.

2.4.4 Exclusion of Alternative Causes of Vestibular Symptoms Besides Migraine

The final step in diagnosing vestibular migraine is to determine whether or not migraine is the only or the best explanation for the correlation between the identified vestibular symptoms and the migraine diagnosis. If the vestibular symptoms are clearly caused by, or are better related to, a recognized vestibular disorder, the diagnosis of vestibular migraine should be questioned. To do so, a careful differential diagnosis is needed and is usually not a significant challenge to an experienced clinician. However, difficulties are often encountered when a possible correlation between the vestibular symptoms and migraine cannot be completely rejected. For example, some migraine patients may also have vestibular symptoms that are clearly or reasonably believed to be not related to migraine. These vestibular symptoms may occur either by coincidence or due to aggravation during or between migraine attacks. In many cases, the underlying cause of vestibular symptoms can be a minor vestibular, visual, or cerebellar dysfunction that is normally asymptomatic but becomes unmasked or exacerbated during migraine attacks. In other words, despite independent mechanisms, vestibular symptoms and migraine may still interact and reciprocally influence each other. Further, a few neurological disorders in the spectrum of migraine can present with prominent vertiginous symptoms. Those disorders can be distinguished from vestibular migraine based on some of their unique clinical features. These conditions will be discussed later in differential diagnosis.

Having made all the above efforts, the gathered findings are examined against the recommended diagnostic criteria for vestibular migraine. A final diagnosis of vestibular migraine can be made if all the requirements are fulfilled [8].

2.4.5 Comments

A few important clinical aspects need to be further discussed. First, the inquiry of medical history should always include asking questions about all the medical conditions that can be relevant to vestibular function, such as cardiac and pulmonary functions, psychiatric and psychological status, childhood development, and, if any, previous diseases that involved peripheral and central nervous systems especially the vestibular system. Women should also be evaluated for their history of menstruation and possible complications with it. Patients should also be routinely asked for current or previous neurological and otological disorders such as motion sickness, gait and balance disorders, visual discomfort, eye misalignment, impaired control of ocular movement, auditory symptoms, head trauma, infection of brain or ear, etc. Relevant social history, such as previous and current medication and substance abuse, and family history, especially about migraine, vertigo, and unsteadiness, should be routinely obtained.

Second, one should keep it in mind that the diagnosis of vestibular migraine is entirely based on the subjective features of relevant clinical symptoms [8]. In other words, the patients with vestibular migraine are not expected to have any significant finding on their physical examination. Although the physical examination is typically normal or unremarkable for the majority of those patients, subtle physical findings, such as brief episodic nystagmus and saccadic tracking, can be recognized during or between attacks of vestibular migraine [26, 27]. These findings are usually considered as benign and can be directly related to migraine. However, investigations are often made in order to prove that they are indeed not attributed to another disorder.

Finally, supplemental investigations in addition to history taking and physical examination are performed in some patients because of their individual conditions. Those clinical investigations include radiology (such as CT and MRI), vestibular laboratory (such as nystagmogram, vestibular evoked myogenic potentials, rotary chair, and posturography), and audiology laboratory (such as audiometry, auditory evoked potentials, and electrocochleogram). When used appropriately, these clinical tests may provide critical information to help with the differential diagnosis.

2.5 The Differential Diagnosis of Vestibular Migraine

When typical vestibular symptoms and migraine history are both identified and their temporal correlations confirmed in an otherwise healthy person with normal physical examination, the diagnosis of vestibular migraine may be not difficult. A diagnosis of vestibular migraine will be questioned if the identified vestibular symptoms can be explained by an alternative cause better than migraine. Meanwhile, ambiguous presentations or variations are often encountered. For example, an individual who presents with clear vestibular symptoms may have never experienced a headache despite having a typical migraine aura and associated phobia and nausea. In situations such as this, the judgment may heavily depend on the clinician's knowledge and experience. In this section, a few vestibular disorders in which the clinical presentations can significantly overlap with vestibular migraine will be discussed.

2.5.1 Benign Paroxysmal Vertigo of Childhood (BPVC)
(See Also Chap. 4)

As first described by Basser in 1964 [6], BPVC is a paroxysmal pediatric disorder that has been regarded as a migraine equivalent, or a precursor of migraine, in children. Together with migraine, BPVC is a common cause of vertigo in pediatric population [28, 29] and the most common cause of episodic vertigo in children between ages 2 and 5 years [30]. It is classified as one of the *childhood periodic syndromes* in ICHD-II. It is defined as a probably heterogeneous disorder with at least five episodic severe vertigo attacks that occur suddenly without warning, last for minutes to hours, and resolve spontaneously in otherwise healthy young children. The disorder has a typical onset younger than 4 years and usually resolves after age 7–8 years [31]. Clinically, the child may suddenly appear frightened, may exhibit pallor, and has to stop playing. The child may also report having a spinning sensation or may be witnessed with nystagmus. The child may also cry, vomit, and stagger during attacks. The neurological examination is usually normal between attacks and so are the encephalogram, vestibular laboratory, and auditory measures between attacks. However, some abnormalities with auditory and vestibular functional tests within a few days after attacks have been reported [32]. A more complete review of this topic is discussed in Chap. 4.

2.5.2 Basilar-Type Migraine

It has been estimated that more than 60 % of patients with basilar-type migraine may experience vertigo during their attacks [8]. Vestibular migraine and basilar-type migraine are different disorders by their definitions and diagnostic criteria. These two disorders can be differentiated from each other by the more complicated focal neurological deficits with basilar-type migraine. Historically, in the development of the concept of vestibular migraine, all patients with vestibular symptoms were thought to manifest basilar-type migraine; see Chap. 3.

In addition to vertigo, patients with basilar-type migraine also describe complicated migraine auras, such as dysarthria, diplopia, binocular and symmetric visual field disturbances, decreased consciousness, ataxia, bilateral paresthesia, tinnitus, and hypacusia [18]. These symptoms are generally considered as manifestations of transient ischemia involving the brainstem, cerebellum, and bilateral posterior hemispheres. Vestibular migraine is much more common in adults than basilar-type migraine that usually affects adolescents and usually resolves by adulthood [3].

2.5.3 Menière's Disease
(See Also Chap. 6)

Menière's disease is an idiopathic syndrome of endolymphatic hydrops [33]. The diagnosis of definite Menière's disease requires fulfillments of all the following criteria: (1) at least two definitive spontaneous episodes of vertigo lasting from 20 min to 24 h, (2) hearing loss on at least one occasion documented by audiometry, (3) tinnitus and ear fullness on the affected side, and (4) exclusion of other causes.

Despite the apparent differences in their pathologies and clinical presentations, a possible link between Menière's disease and vestibular migraine has been suggested [34]. Migraine has been found to be more common than usual in patients with Menière's disease [3, 35]. Those two conditions may be even genetically related [15, 36, 37]. Similar symptoms, such as vertigo, headache, phobia, and even alternation of hearing, may present in both disorders [38]. Migraine may also facilitate the development of Menière's disease [36]. The differentiation between Menière's disease and vestibular migraine can be difficult when Menière's disease presents with predominantly vestibular symptoms. However, its association with significant fullness and pressure, roaring tinnitus, and progressive sensorineural hearing loss in the affected ear is not the characteristics of migraine.

2.5.4 Benign Paroxysmal Positional Vertigo (BPPV)

Vestibular migraine may present with prominent positional vertigo that can be confused with BPPV. Migraine has been found to be more common in patients with idiopathic BPPV than those with BPPV secondary to other causes [3, 39]. In BPPV, the stereotype association of characteristic spinning vertigo and nystagmus with specific head position leads to a localization at the peripheral vestibular end organ. The absence of intense migraine features and the brief duration of vertigo with each episode lasting only for seconds favor the diagnosis of BPPV rather than vestibular migraine. Many references, including comprehensive review articles [40], are available for the diagnosis of BPPV. The definitive finding of rotary nystagmus when performing the Dix-Hallpike test confirms the diagnosis of BPPV.

2.5.5 Psychiatric Dizziness

The association of migraine with some psychiatric disorders, such as anxiety, panic attacks, and depression, has been well recognized [19–21]. Vestibular symptoms and signs are common in patients with anxiety [41]. Patients with vestibular migraine often also suffer from anxiety [23, 42]. Furman et al. [22] has described a disorder named *migraine-anxiety-related dizziness (MARD)* which is a combination of dizziness, migraine, and anxiety.

2.5.6 Motion Sickness

Motion sickness refers to a combination of symptoms and signs that reflect an individual's cognitive and autonomic dysfunction in response to a certain type of environmental motion [3, 43]. Symptoms related to motion sickness, such as cognitive cloudiness, wooziness or dizziness, nausea, vomiting, unsteadiness, headaches, and diaphoresis, are similar to vestibular migraine [44]. Individuals with migraine, especially vestibular migraine, are more susceptible to motion sickness [3, 45, 46]. As a result, these two conditions often occur together in many individuals. In clinical practice, the diagnosis of motion sickness is usually not difficult. However, one should be aware of its overlaps with migraine and the subsequent comorbidities when either migraine or motion sickness is suspected.

2.5.7 Mal de Debarquement Syndrome (MdD)

MdD is characterized by the persistent sensation of motion as if the individual were still on board a ship after the person has disembarked. Symptoms associated with this disorder include persistent rocking, swaying, imbalance, poor concentration, visual disturbances, ear fullness, hyperacusis, and fatigue [47, 48]. Maladaptive neuroplasticity has been proposed as the mechanism for MdD [47]. It has been reported that migraine patients are more likely to develop MdD than those without migraine [48].

2.5.8 Familial Hemiplegic Migraine (FHM)

FHM is a type of migraine with aura according to the ICHD-II [18]. It is also regarded as a complicated migraine type because of the transient neurological deficits such as hemiplegia during its typical attacks. Progress has been made to uncover the genetic basis of this autosomal dominant hereditary disease of which several types have been identified [5]. Mutations of CACNA1A gene on chromosome 19, which codes for the α1A subunit of voltage-gated P/Q-type calcium channels, have been identified in families with FHM1. The same genetic mutation is found with episodic ataxia type

2 and spinocerebellar ataxia type 6. Mutation of ATP1A2 gene on chromosome 1, which codes for Na/K-ATPase, is linked to FHM2. Mutation of the SCN1A gene, which codes for α subunit of sodium channel, has been linked to FHM3 [49, 50]. Differentiating these hereditary conditions from vestibular migraine can be difficult as a family history may be present in both conditions and genetic testing is often not clinically practical. It is possible that some potentially independent disorders may be currently under the subjective diagnosis of vestibular migraine.

2.5.9 Other Episodic and Paroxysmal Vestibular Disorders That May Mimic Migraine

Vestibular paroxysmia results from irritation of vestibular nerve by surrounding cerebral arteries, usually a branch of anterior inferior cerebral artery, close to or inside the internal auditory canal. *Transient ischemic attacks* in the vertebrobasilar arterial territory may cause vestibular symptoms and signs when the ischemia has affected peripheral or central vestibular structures. *Chronic subjective dizziness (CSD)* sometimes can be also confused with migraine as both may present with similar symptoms such as unsteadiness, dizziness, and motion intolerance [51]. In general, CSD is typically non-vertiginous.

Conclusion

Vestibular migraine is common. The diagnosis of vestibular migraine is based on the conclusion that an individual's vestibular symptoms cannot be better attributed to any other disorder other than migraine. The clinician needs to first identify symptoms of truly vestibular etiology in a patient with a clear history of migraine, then to confirm the presence of a correlation between the vestibular symptoms and migraine, and finally to justify that migraine is more appropriate than other disorders to cause these symptoms. Until our understanding about this condition has been further advanced, the entire diagnostic process will be purely subjective.

The recently proposed criteria to define vestibular symptoms and to diagnose vestibular migraine by the Bárány Society and the International Headache Society can be used to guide clinical practice. According to these criteria, a diagnosis of vestibular migraine can be made when the appropriate number of vestibular attacks occurs in patients who have a history of migraine and experience either headaches typical of migraine, or photophobia and phonophobia, or migraine aura at least with 50 % of their vestibular attacks. *Possible* vestibular migraine can be diagnosed in patients with vestibular symptoms and *either* a prior history of migraine headaches *or* symptoms of headaches typical of migraine, or photophobia and phonophobia, or migraine aura at least with 50 % of their vestibular attacks.

References

1. Neuhauser H, Leopold M, von Brevern M, Arnold G, Lempert T. The interrelations of migraine, vertigo, and migrainous vertigo. Neurology. 2001;56(4):436–41.
2. Neuhauser HK, Radtke A, von Brevern M, Feldmann M, Lezius F, Ziese T, Lempert T. Migrainous vertigo: prevalence and impact on quality of life. Neurology. 2006;67:1028–33.
3. Furman JM, Marcus D. Migraine and motion sensitivity. Contin Lifelong Learn Neurol. 2012;18(5):1102–17.
4. Rothrock JF. Understanding migraine: a tale of hope and frustration. Headache. 2011;51(7):1188–90.
5. Ward TN. Migraine diagnosis and pathophysiology. Contin Lifelong Learn Neurol. 2012;18(4):753–63.
6. Basser LS. Benign paroxysmal vertigo of childhood: a variety of vestibular neuronitis. Brain. 1964;87:141–52.
7. Lempert T. Vestibular migraine. Semin Neurol. 2013;33:212–8.
8. Lempert T, Olesen J, Furman J, Waterston J, Seemungal B, Carey J, Bisdorff A, Versino M, Evers S, Newman-Toker D. Vestibular migraine: diagnostic criteria – consensus document of the Barany Society and the International Headache Society. J Vestib Res. 2012;22:167–72.
9. Halmagyi GC, Baloh RW. Chapter 23. Overview of common syndromes of vestibular disease. In: Baloh RW, Halmagyi GC, editors. Disorders of the vestibular system. New York: Oxford University Press; 1996. p. 291–9.
10. Bisdorff A, Von Brevern M, Lempert T, Newman-Toker DE. Classification of vestibular symptoms:

towards an international classification of vestibular disorders. J Vestib Res. 2009;19:1–13.

11. Dieterich M. Central vestibular disorders. J Neurol. 2007;254:559–68.

12. Balaban CD. Migraine, vertigo and migrainous vertigo: links between vestibular and pain mechanisms. J Vestib Res. 2011;21(6):315–21.

13. Lee H, Sohn SL, Jung DK, et al. Migraine and isolated recurrent vertigo of unknown cause. Neurol Res. 2002;24(7):663–5.

14. Cha YH, Lee H, Santell LS, Baloh RW. Association of benign recurrent vertigo and migraine in 208 patients. Celphalalgia. 2009;29(5):550–5.

15. Cha YH. Migraine-associated vertigo: diagnosis and treatment. Semin Neurol. 2010;30(2):167–74.

16. Lempert T, Neuhauser H. Epidemiology of vertigo, migraine and vestibular migraine. J Neurol. 2009;256: 333–8.

17. Cherian N. Vertigo as a migraine phenomenon. Curr Neurol Neurosci Rep. 2013;13:343. pp 1–6.

18. International Headache Society Classification Subcommittee. International classification of headache disorders. 2nd edition. Cephalalgia. 2004;24 Suppl 1: 1–160.

19. Breslau N, Davis GC, Andreski P. Migraine, psychiatric disorders, and suicide attempts: an epidemiologic study of young adults. Psychiatry Res. 1991;37:11–23.

20. Breslau N, Schultz LR, Stewart WF, Lipton RB, Lucia VC, Welch KM. Headache and major depression: is the association specific to migraine? Neurology. 2000; 54:308–13.

21. Breslau N, Schultz LR, Stewart WF, Lipton R, Welch KMA. Headache types and panic disorder. Directionality and specificity. Neurology. 2001;56:350–4.

22. Furman JM, Balaban CD, Jacob RG, Marcus D. Migraine-anxiety related dizziness (MARD): a new disorder? J Neurol Neurosurg Psychiatry. 2005;76(1):1–8.

23. Best C, Eckhardt-Henn A, Tschan R, Dieterich M. Psychiatric morbidity and comorbidity in different vestibular vertigo syndromes. Results of a prospective longitudinal study over one year. J Neurol. 2009;256(1):58–65.

24. Eggers SD, Zee DS. Evaluating the dizzy patient: bedside examination and laboratory assessment of the vestibular system. Semin Neurol. 2003;23(1):47–58.

25. Newman-Toker DE. Symptoms and signs of neuro-otologic disorders. Contin Lifelong Learn Neurol. 2012;18(5):1016–40.

26. von Brevern M, Zeise D, Neuhauser H, Clarke AH, Lempert T. Acute migrainous vertigo: clinical and oculographic findings. Brain. 2005;128(Pt 2):365–74.

27. Radtke A, von Brevern M, Neuhauser H, Hottenrott T, Lempert T. Vestibular migraine: long-term follow-up of clinical symptoms and vestibulo-cochlear findings. Neurology. 2012;79(15):1607–14.

28. Erbek SH, Erbek SS, Yilmaz I, Topal O, Ozgirgin N, Ozluoglu LN, Alehan F. Vertigo in childhood: a clinical experience. Int J Pediatr Otorhinolaryngol. 2006;70: 1547–54.

29. Gioacchini FM, Alicandri-Ciufelli M, Kaleci S, Magliulo G, Re M. Prevalence and diagnosis of vestibular disorders in children: a review. Int J Pediatr Otorhinolaryngol. 2014;78:718–24.

30. Langhagen T, Schroeder AS, Rettinger N, Borggraefe I, Klaus J. Migraine-related vertigo and somatoform vertigo frequently occur in children and are often associated. Neuropediatrics. 2013;44(1):55–8.

31. Baloh RW. Neurotology of migraine. Headache. 1997; 37:615–21.

32. Zhang D, Fan Z, Han Y, Wang M, Xu L, Luo J, Ai Y, Wang H. Benign paroxysmal vertigo of childhood: diagnostic value of vestibular test and high stimulus rate auditory brainstem response test. Int J Pediatr Otorhinolaryngol. 2012;76:107–10.

33. Committee on Hearing and Equilibrium. Committee on hearing and equilibrium guidelines for the diagnosis and evaluation of therapy in Meniere's disease. Otolaryngol Head Neck Surg. 1995;113:181–5.

34. Murofushi T, Ozeki H, Inoue A, Sakata A. Does migraine-associated vertigo share a common pathophysiology with Meniere's disease? Study with vestibular-evoked myogenic potential. Cephalalgia. 2009;29(12): 1259–66.

35. Radtke A, Lempert T, Gresty MA, Brookes GB, Bronstein AM, Neuhauser H. Migraine and Ménière's disease: is there a link? Neurology. 2002;59:1700–4.

36. Cha YH, Brodsky J, Ishiyama G, Sabatti C, Baloh RW. The relevance of migraine in patients with Ménière's disease. Acta Otolaryngol. 2007;127: 1241–5.

37. Cha YH, Kane MJ, Baloh RW. Familial clustering of migraine, episodic vertigo, and Ménière's disease. Otol Neurotol. 2008;29:93–6.

38. Brantberg K, Baloh RW. Similarity of vertigo attacks due to Meniere's disease and benign recurrent vertigo both with and without migraine. Acta Otolaryngol. 2011;131:722–7.

39. Ishiyama A, Jacobson KM, Baloh RW. Migraine and benign positional vertigo. Ann Otol Rhinol Laryngol. 2000;109:377–80.

40. Fife TD. Positional dizziness. Contin Lifelong Learn Neurol. 2012;18(5):1060–85.

41. Margraf J, Taylor B, Ehlers A, Roth WT, Agras WS. Panic attacks in the natural environment. J Nerv Ment Dis. 1987;175:558–65.

42. Salhofer S, Lieba-Samal D, Freydl E, Bartl S, Wiest G, Wöber C. Migraine and vertigo – a prospective diary study. Cephalalgia. 2010;30(7):821–8.

43. Money KE. Motion sickness. Physiol Rev. 1970;50(1): 1–39.

44. Graybiel A, Wood CD, Miller EF, Cramer DB. Diagnostic criteria for grading the severity of acute motion sickness. Aerosp Med. 1968;39(5):453–5.

45. Marcus DA, Furman JM, Balaban CD. Motion sickness in migraine sufferers. Expert Opin Pharmacother. 2005;6:2691–7.

46. Cuomo-Granston A, Drummond PD. Migraine and motion sickness: what is the link? Prog Neurobiol. 2010;91(4):300–12.

47. Gordon CR, Spitzer O, Doweck I, Melamed Y, Shupak A. Clinical features of mal de debarquement:

adaptation and habituation to sea conditions. J Vestib Res. 1995;5:363–9.

48. Cha YH, Brodsky J, Ishiyama G, Sabatti C, Baloh RW. Clinical features and associated syndromes of mal de debarquement. J Neurol. 2008;255(7):1038–44.

49. Von Brevern M, Ta N, Shankar A, Wiste A, Siegel A, Radtke A, Sander T, Escayg A. Migrainous vertigo: mutation analysis of the candidate genes CACNA1A, ATP1A2, SCN1A, and CACNB4. Headache. 2006;46(7):1136–41.

50. Lee H, Jen JC, Cha YH, et al. Phenotypic and genetic analysis of a large family with migraine-associated vertigo. Headache. 2008;48(10):1460–7.

51. Staab JP. Chronic subjective dizziness. Contin Lifelong Learn Neurol. 2012;18(5):1118–41.

Historical Perspective of Vestibular Migraine

3

Joseph M. Furman and Carey D. Balaban

3.1 History of Medicine Perspective

The accounts of vertigo and migraine-like disorders in the ancient literature are highly consistent with the current view that vestibular migraine is a migraine variant produced by the convergence of vestibular information within migraine circuits [1], in a manner similar to auditory, visual, and somesthetic information. In the Hippocratic corpus, vertigo was regarded as a disease of the head, which could be (1) a symptom of engorgement of the head with blood [2] or (2) comorbid with fever, a throbbing head, and thin urine, with the notation that vertigo sufferers with headache tend to show madness [3]. Aretæus of Cappodocia (first century of the Common Era) includes vertigo (1) as a separate chronic disease, (2) as a symptom of a form of the Cephalæa, the hetero-

c*rania* (migraine), and (3) as a prognostic in some individuals for melancholia, epilepsy, or mania [4]. There is little doubt that Cephalæa includes migraine, from its later description as "... an extreme paine in the heed, that a man can nat abide no lyght nor no noyse, and the patient doth loue to be in darke places. And his heed he dothe thynke doth go in peces, and a pylowe is better for the pacient, than a cote of defence [5]." "Vertigo or giddiness" and "hemicrania or megrim" were presented in successive chapters in the works of Ambrose Paré, with similar etiologic descriptions [6]. This association persisted into the early twentieth century. For example, Lectures I and II of Gowers' Clinical Lectures on the Borderland of Epilepsy discussed vertigo [7, 8], followed by Lecture III on migraine [9]. The first use of the term vestibular migraine by Boenheim was discussed within this framework of clinical similarities between vertigo, migraine, and epilepsy [10].

3.2 Modern Era Perspective of Vestibular Migraine

More than 50 years ago, Selby and Lance [11] published a paper regarding the clinical aspects of 500 patients with migraine and what was then called vascular headache. These authors noted that vertigo occurred in 33 % of these patients during headache. Although the pathophysiology of this symptom was uncertain, this large series

J.M. Furman, MD, PhD (✉)
Departments of Otolaryngology, Neurology,
Bioengineering and Physical Therapy,
University of Pittsburgh, Eye and Ear Institute Suite
500, 200 Lothrop Street, Pittsburgh, PA 15213, USA
e-mail: furmanjm@upmc.edu

C.D. Balaban, PhD
Departments of Otolaryngology, Neurobiology,
Communication Science & Disorders, and
Bioengineering, University of Pittsburgh,
Eye and Ear Institute, Suite 107, 200 Lothrop Street,
Pittsburgh, PA 15213, USA
e-mail: cbalaban@upmc.edu

S. Wetmore, A. Rubin (eds.), *Vestibular Migraine*,
DOI 10.1007/978-3-319-14550-1_3, © Springer International Publishing Switzerland 2015

23

of patients provided clear evidence for an association between vestibular symptoms and migraine and confirmed previous observations by Boenheim [10], Heveroch [12], Symonds [13], Richter [14], and Friedman et al. [15] of dizziness symptoms during headache. In 1961, Bickerstaff described the so-called basilar artery migraine, now known as "basilar-type migraine," as a disorder in which vestibular symptoms, including vertigo, are often prominent [16]. Sturzenegger and Meienberg reported that 63 % of such patients had vertigo [17]. However, only a small percentage of patients who meet the current criteria for vestibular migraine also meet criteria for basilar artery migraine [18]. Bickerstaff's 1961 description firmly established vestibular symptoms as a component of the symptomatology of some patients with migraine headache.

The idea that vestibular symptoms could be a migraine equivalent independent of headache was suggested earlier by Heveroch [12], Symonds [13], Richter [14], and Levy and O'Leary [19]. Vestibular symptoms independent of headache were not generally considered as a possible migrainous phenomenon. Fenichel's 1967 paper [20] proposed that "benign paroxysmal vertigo of childhood," described initially by Basser in 1964 [21], was a migraine variant seen in childhood. More than 10 years later, Slater's 1979 paper [22] proposed a link between "benign recurrent vertigo" in adults and migraine. Kuritzky et al. described 84 patients with migraine [23] and found that vestibular symptoms and signs, such as vertigo and dizziness, were more common in migraine than in controls. These authors also found that vestibular laboratory abnormalities are common in patients with migraine [24]. These authors noted that vestibular symptoms occurred both temporally associated with migraine headache and interictally, i.e., between headaches, thereby furthering the concept that vestibular symptoms can be a migraine equivalent.

A link between vestibular abnormalities and migraine was confirmed by the landmark paper by Kayan and Hood in 1984 [25]. They noted a high prevalence of vestibular problems in patients with migraine headache as compared with patients with tension-type headache. Although not the first paper that identified the link between migraine and vestibular symptoms, nearly every paper regarding vestibular migraine since 1984 cites the Kayan and Hood paper as establishing a link between vestibular abnormalities and migraine in adults. Harker, in 1987 [26], proposed a classification scheme for grading the likelihood of an etiological rather than chance association between vestibular symptoms and migraine using the terms definite, probable, and possible. Some years later, Parker [27] emphasized the concept that paroxysmal vertigo occurred in patients with migraine and that the key observation regarding the association between migraine and vestibular symptoms is the temporal relationship between dizziness and headache. Parker noted that this temporal relationship can be quite variable.

Cutrer and Baloh in 1992 [28] were the first to introduce a series of papers that addressed the link between migraine and vestibular symptoms in patients who presented with dizziness rather than headache. Cutrer and Baloh coined the term "migraine-associated dizziness" to describe a small number of patients, i.e., 91 of 5,000 patients, who were seen for dizziness in a tertiary care setting, whose symptoms could not be attributed to an alternative disorder and who suffered from migraine. Sixty-nine percent of these patients had vertigo. There was a wide range of duration of symptoms with about half of the patient's reporting dizziness symptoms lasting for more than 1 day. Further support for a link between migraine and vestibular symptoms was provided in 1993 by Aragones et al. [29] who reported a high prevalence (about 33 %) of migraine in a group of 72 patients with vertigo of uncertain cause. In 1997, Savundra et al. coined the term "migraine-associated vertigo" [30]. These authors also noted a high prevalence (about 32 %) of migraine in a group of 363 patients with vertigo and advocated for migraine-associated vertigo to be considered a distinct diagnostic entity. In that same year, Cass et al. [31] described 100 patients out of a total population of 4,400 who had a condition they termed "migraine-related vestibulopathy." These authors considered migraine-related vestibulopathy as a distinct diagnostic entity and described laboratory abnormalities in this group. The diagnosis of migraine-related vestibulopathy was based on a combination of migraine headache, space and motion discomfort [32], and no other better diagnosis. By this time, migraine-related dizziness was considered a diagnostic possibility in all patients with dizziness whose signs and symptoms could not be ascribed to another recognizable neurotologic syndrome.

Johnson, in 1998 [33], provided a retrospective description of the clinical findings in a group of 99 of 665 patients with migraine-related dizziness/migraine-related vertigo using the diagnostic criteria that patients needed to have both migraine and dizziness/vertigo without a better diagnosis. Johnson's contribution was primarily to promote the idea that treatment of these patients for migraine yielded favorable outcomes. This finding suggested that migraine-related dizziness was a bona fide disorder for which there was efficacious treatment and motivated the medical community to establish migraine-related dizziness as a diagnostic entity because of the possibility of successful treatment. In 1999, Dieterich and Brandt [34] published a highly regarded paper that reintroduced the term "vestibular migraine," a designation first used by Boenheim [10] in 1917. Dieterich and Brandt [34] highlighted the concept that vestibular migraine is distinct from basilar-type migraine and that objective vestibular abnormalities are commonly seen between episodes of dizziness. Shortly thereafter, in 2001, Neuhauser et al. [35], in a seminal paper, established diagnostic criteria for a condition they termed "migrainous vertigo," which has subsequently been renamed "vestibular migraine." Neuhauser et al. [35] found that the lifetime prevalence of vestibular migraine was 7 % in their population of 200 patients with dizziness. A follow-on paper some 10 years later confirmed the validity of the Neuhauser diagnostic criteria for vestibular migraine [36]. Subsequent papers confirmed the clinical utility of considering a diagnosis of vestibular migraine. In 2002, Reploeg and Goebel [37] reported a 72 % rate of efficacy of anti-migrainous therapy in a group of 81 patients with vestibular migraine.

In 2011, Strupp et al. [38] outlined detailed treatment options for vestibular migraine noting that "vestibular migraine is increasingly regarded as the most common central cause of recurrent attacks of vertigo." The diagnostic criteria for vestibular migraine published in 2012 [39], which are based upon a consensus between the Barany Society and the International Headache Society, firmly established vestibular migraine as a diagnostic entity. Now that there is general agreement upon nomenclature and diagnostic criteria, the field can focus on studies of the pathophysiology and management of vestibular migraine.

3.3   Origins of Current Diagnostic Criteria for Vestibular Migraine

With the acceptance of diagnostic criteria for vestibular migraine [39], there is some interest in reviewing the origins of these criteria. The term "vestibular migraine" was used initially by Boenheim in the early 1900s [10] in his description of patients with vertigo and migraine. As the association between vestibular symptoms and migraine was becoming recognized, various terms were used to describe what in retrospect was probably the same diagnostic entity, namely, what we now call vestibular migraine. The term "basilar artery migraine" was introduced by Bickerstaff in 1961 [16] to describe a type of migraine that often was associated with vestibular symptoms. Sturzenegger and Meienberg in 1985 [17] noted that 63 % of patients with confirmed basilar artery migraine complained of vertigo. The term "basilar-type migraine" replaced the term basilar artery migraine [40] and remains in usage to describe a type of migraine that may be associated with vestibular symptoms. However, few patients who meet diagnostic criteria for vestibular migraine also meet criteria for basilar-type migraine [18], which highlighted the need for a specific diagnostic entity that recognizes the large number of patients with migraine-related vestibular symptoms who lacked a diagnosis.

The terms "benign paroxysmal vertigo of childhood" [21] and "benign recurrent vertigo" [22] for adults also were used to denote a condition akin to vestibular migraine highlighting the episodic nature of the condition. Other terms such as "migraine-associated dizziness" [28], "migraine-associated vertigo" [30], "migraine-related vestibulopathy" [31], and "migrainous vertigo" [35] have each had their proponents. Dieterich and Brandt in 1999 [34] reintroduced the term "vestibular migraine," which is the nomenclature that is now agreed upon by both the Barany Society and the International Headache Society. Prior to the Neuhauser et al. 2001 seminal paper [35], there were no firm diagnostic criteria for vestibular migraine. For the most part, vestibular migraine was given different names and in its various forms, was considered a diagnosis of exclusion and was ascribed to patients without a definitive neurotologic diagnosis such as Meniere's disease or BPPV, who suffered from migraine. The absence of strict diagnostic criteria resulted in a high degree of variability in estimates of incidence and prevalence and precluded reliable meta-analyses and treatment trials. Since 2001, most studies of vestibular migraine have used the Neuhauser et al. 2001 [35] criteria, which were validated in a 2012 study that reassessed the initial cohort of patients regarding their current diagnosis [41]. Brandt and Strupp in 2010 [42] described treatment options for what is now considered an established diagnostic entity. The diagnostic criteria for vestibular migraine published in 2012 [39] were minimally different from those proposed by Neuhauser et al. in 2001 [35]. Importantly, these latest criteria were based on an international consensus of neurologists and otolaryngologists and were consistent with diagnostic criteria for migraine and its variants established by the International Headache Society [40]. The establishment of diagnostic criteria for vestibular migraine should pave the way for future studies of the epidemiology, pathophysiology, and treatment of this now widely recognized, common, neurotologic disorder.

3.4 Pathophysiologic Perspective

The clinical evidence of comorbidity and advances in studies of migraine mechanisms suggested an overarching hypothesis that central vestibular pathways and the inner ear share the vascular, neurogenic inflammation and central neural mechanisms that have been implicated in the pathogenesis of migraine [43–47]. The development of this approach may be traced sequentially in review papers [1, 48–52]. Hence, vestibular migraine can be regarded as a migraine variant with vestibular manifestations.

The vascular theory of migraine was developed in the late 1930s by Harold Wolff [53, 54]. He proposed that preheadache phenomena (including vertigo) were the result of oligemia and/or transient ischemia from vasoconstriction. The headache pain, by contrast, was proposed to result from a rebound vasodilation and consequent activation of trigeminal nociceptors. Bickerstaff's (1961) [16] concept of "basilar artery migraine" (or "basilar-type migraine") was a logical extension of this model to involvement of vertebrobasilar perfusion of the vestibular nuclei, nerve, and inner ear. An expanded trigeminocerebrovascular system [55] concept provided a focus for exploring the link between vascular responsiveness and pain as a physiological consequence of activation of trigeminal ganglion innervation of cerebral and meningeal vasculature. Because the trigeminovascular system also innervates blood supply of the inner ear [56, 57], the concept was also consistent with a role in the known sensitivity to sound and vertigo in migraine.

More recent extensions of vascular theories of migraine include Iadecola's [58] hypothesis about the role of neurovascular interactions in migraine. He suggested that the extracellular release of neocortical signal substrates (e.g., K^+, H^+, arachidonic acid, and nitric oxide) during cortical spreading depression would activate trigeminal afferents on cranial blood vessels. These afferents would then elicit a trigeminovascular reflex-mediated vasodilation in the meninges, via a parasympathetic relay in the sphenopalatine ganglion. Simultaneously, as described by Moskowitz [45], peptide secretion from axon collaterals of the trigeminal ganglion cells (an "axon reflex") would elicit a sterile inflammatory response in meningeal vessels. Parallel phenomena occur in the inner ear [59, 60]. Because the vasodilation is neither necessary nor sufficient for perception of headache pain [47, 55, 58, 61], migraine headache pain is now attributed primarily to central processing of the trigeminal afferent activation in ascending thalamocortical pathways [44, 47, 58]. However, it seems prudent to reserve judgment before rejecting the possibility that vasodilation can contribute to migraine headache pain [62] or vestibular migraine.

Ho et al. [44] expanded the "migraine circuit" concept from strictly trigeminal pathways for vascular regulation and pain perception to a framework that includes central circuits for triggers and premonitory symptoms. The external trigger circuits include visual, auditory, somatosensory, and chemical (olfactory and gustatory) sensory pathways. Internal triggers include hormonal fluctuations and stress, which can be defined for migraine as "environmental factors or demands that may be perceived as demanding or negative" [63]. Both internal and external triggers involve structures such as the hypothalamus and amygdala, which show altered activity associated with migraine [64–68]. Vestibular pathways can be viewed as integral components of these migraine circuits. The fact that components of the "migraine circuit" are activated during induction of vestibular-induced motion sickness [69] indicates that vestibular migraine is an indicator of the more widespread role of vestibular information processing in sensory, motor, and affective domains.

In conclusion, the evolution of the recognition of vestibular migraine as a distinct neurotologic diagnosis represents a fascinating progression from obscurity to wide acceptance. Hopefully, by understanding how such a transformation could occur, clinicians will be better able to care for patients with vestibular migraine and remain open-minded regarding other poorly understood disorders.

References

1. Furman JM, Marcus DA, Balaban CD. Vestibular migraine: clinical aspects and pathophysiology. Lancet Neurol. 2013;12:706–15.
2. Potter P. Hippocrates, vol. V. Cambridge: Harvard University Press; 1988. p. 196–7.
3. Potter P. Hippocrates, vol. VI. Cambridge: Harvard University Press; 1988. p. 280–1.
4. Adams F. The extant works of Aretæus, the Cappodocian. London: The Sydenham Society; 1856.
5. Borde A. The Breuiary of Helthe, for all maner of syckenesses and diseases the which may be in man, or woman doth folowe. Amsterdam: Da Capo Press; 1971.
6. Johnson T. The workes of that famous chirurgion Ambrose Parey translated out of Latine and compared with the French. London: T. Cotes and R. Young; 1634.
7. Gowers WR. Clinical lectures on the borderland of epilepsy: vertigo. Br Med J. 1906;2:7–11.
8. Gowers WR. Clinical lectures ON THE BORDERLAND OF EPILEPSY: VERTIGO: Delivered at the National Hospital for the Paralysed and Epileptic. Br Med J. 1906;2:128–31.
9. Gowers WR. Clinical lectures on the borderland of epilepsy: III. Migraine. Br Med J. 1906;2:1617–22.
10. Boenheim F. Über familiare Hemicrania vestibularis. Neurol Zentralbl. 1917;36:226–9.
11. Selby G, Lance JW. Observations on 500 cases of migraine and allied vascular headache. J Neurol Neurosurg Psychiatry. 1960;23:23–32.
12. Heveroch J. La migraine vestibulaire. Rev Neurol. 1925;33:925–9.
13. Symonds CP. Vertigo. Postgrad Med J. 1926;1:63–5.
14. Richter H. Die Migrane *Handbuch der Neurologie*. Berlin: Springer; 1935. p. 166–245.
15. Friedman AP, Von Storch TJ, Merritt HH. Migraine and tension headaches; a clinical study of two thousand cases. Neurology. 1954;4:773–88.
16. Bickerstaff ER. Basilar artery migraine. Lancet. 1961;227:15–7.
17. Sturzenegger MH, Meienberg O. Basilar artery migraine: a follow-up study of 82 cases. Headache. 1985;25:408–15.
18. Eggers SD. Migraine-related vertigo: diagnosis and treatment. Curr Pain Headache Rep. 2007;11:217–26.
19. Levy I, O'Leary JL. Incidence of vertigo in neurological conditions. Ann Otol Rhinol Laryngol. 1947;56:557–75.
20. Fenichel GM. Migraine as a cause of benign paroxysmal vertigo of childhood. J Pediatr. 1967;71:114–5.
21. Basser LS. Benign paroxysmal vertigo of childhood. (a variety of vestibular neuronitis). Brain J Neurol. 1964;87:141–52.
22. Slater R. Benign recurrent vertigo. J Neurol Neurosurg Psychiatry. 1979;42:363–7.
23. Kuritzky A, Ziegler DK, Hassanein R. Vertigo, motion sickness and migraine. Headache. 1981;21:227–31.

24. Kuritzky A, Toglia UJ, Thomas D. Vestibular function in migraine. Headache. 1981;21:110–2.
25. Kayan A, Hood JD. Neuro-otological manifestations of migraine. Brain J Neurol. 1984;107:1123–42.
26. Harker LA, Rassekh CH. Episodic vertigo in basilar artery migraine. Otolaryngol Head Neck Surg. 1987;96:239–50.
27. Parker W. Migraine and the vestibular system in adults. Am J Otol. 1991;12:25–34.
28. Cutrer FM, Baloh RW. Migraine-associated dizziness. Headache. 1992;32:300–4.
29. Aragones JM, Fortes-Rego J, Fuste J, Cardozo A. Migraine: an alternative in the diagnosis of unclassified vertigo. Headache. 1993;33:125–8.
30. Savundra PA, Carroll JD, Davies RA, Luxon LM. Migraine-associated vertigo. Cephalalgia. 1997;17:505–10; discussion 487.
31. Cass SP, Furman JM, Ankerstjerne K, Balaban C, Yetiser S, Aydogan B. Migraine-related vestibulopathy. Ann Otol Rhinol Laryngol. 1997;106:182–9.
32. Lilienfeld SO, Jacob RG, Furman JM. Vestibular dysfunction followed by panic disorder with agoraphobia. J Nerv Ment Dis. 1989;177:700–1.
33. Johnson GD. Medical management of migraine-related dizziness and vertigo. Laryngoscope. 1998;108:1–28.
34. Dieterich M, Brandt T. Episodic vertigo related to migraine (90 cases): vestibular migraine? J Neurol. 1999;246:883–92.
35. Neuhauser H, Leopold M, von Brevern M, Arnold G, Lempert T. The interrelations of migraine, vertigo, and migrainous vertigo. Neurology. 2001;56:436–41.
36. Radtke A, Neuhauser H, von Brevern M, Hottenrott T, Lempert T. Vestibular migraine–validity of clinical diagnostic criteria. Cephalalgia. 2011;31:906–13.
37. Reploeg MD, Goebel JA. Migraine-associated dizziness: patient characteristics and management options. Otol Neurotol. 2002;23:364–71.
38. Strupp M, Thurtell MJ, Shaikh AG, Brandt T, Zee DS, Leigh RJ. Pharmacotherapy of vestibular and ocular motor disorders, including nystagmus. J Neurol. 2011;258:1207–22.
39. Lempert T, Olesen J, Furman J, et al. Vestibular migraine: diagnostic criteria. J Vestib Res. 2012;22:167–72.
40. Headache Classification Subcommittee of the International Headache Society. The international classification of headache disorders: 2nd edition. Cephalalgia. 2004;24 Suppl 1:9–160.
41. Radtke A, von Brevern M, Neuhauser H, Hottenrott T, Lempert T. Vestibular migraine: long-term follow-up of clinical symptoms and vestibulo-cochlear findings. Neurology. 2012;79:1607–14.
42. Brandt T, Strupp M. Clicking the eye muscles? The diagnostic value of sound-evoked vestibular reflexes. Neurology. 2010;75:848–9.
43. Goadsby PJ, Lipton RB, Ferrari MD. Drug therapy: migraine–current understanding and treatment. N Engl J Med. 2002;346:257–70.
44. Ho TW, Edvinsson L, Goadsby PJ. CGRP and its receptors provide new insights in migraine pathophysiology. Nat Rev Neurol. 2010;6:573–82.
45. Moskowitz MA. Neurogenic inflammation in the pathophysiology and treatment of migraine. Neurology. 1993;43:S16–20.
46. Moskowitz MA. Pathophysiology of headache–past and present. Headache. 2007;47 Suppl 1:S58–63.
47. Pietrobon D, Striessnig J. Neurobiology of migraine. Nat Rev Neurosci. 2003;4:387–98.
48. Furman JM, Marcus DA, Balaban CD. Migrainous vertigo: development of a pathogenetic model and structured diagnostic interview. Curr Opin Neurol. 2003;16:5–13.
49. Furman JM, Balaban CD, Jacob RG, Marcus DA. Migraine-anxiety related dizziness (MARD): a new disorder? J Neurol Neurosurg Psychiatry. 2005;76:1–8.
50. Marcus DA, Furman JM, Balaban CD. Motion sickness in migraine sufferers. Expert Opin Pharmacother. 2005;6:2691–7.
51. Balaban CD, Jacob RG, Furman JM. Neurologic bases for comorbidity of balance disorders, anxiety disorders and migraine: neurotherapeutic implications. Expert Rev Neurother. 2011;11:379–94.
52. Balaban CD. Migraine, vertigo and migrainous vertigo: Links between vestibular and pain mechanisms. J Vestib Res. 2011;21:315–21.
53. Wolff HG. Headache and other head pain. New York: Oxford University Press; 1948.
54. Graham JR, Wolff HG. Mechanism of migraine headache and action of ergotamine tartrate. AMA Arch Neurol Psychiatry. 1938;39:737–63.
55. May A, Goadsby PJ. The trigeminovascular system in humans: pathophysiologic implications for primary headache syndromes of the neural influences on the cerebral circulation. J Cereb Blood Flow Metab. 1999;19:115–27.
56. Vass Z, Dai CF, Steyger PS, Jancsó G, Trune DR, Nuttall AL. Co-localization of the vanilloid capsaicin receptor and substance P in sensory nerve fibers innervating cochlear and vertebro-basilar arteries. Neuroscience. 2004;124:919–27.
57. Vass Z, Shore SE, Nuttall AL, Miller JM. Direct evidence of trigeminal innervation of cochlear blood vessels. Neuroscience. 1998;84:559–67.
58. Iadecola C. From CSD to headache: a long and winding road. Nat Med. 2002;8:110–2.
59. Koo J-W, Balaban CD. Serotonin-induced plasma extravasation in the murine inner ear: possible mechanism of migraine-associated inner ear dysfunction. Cephalagia. 2006;26:1310–9.
60. Vass Z, Steyger PS, Hordichok AJ, Trune DR, Jancsó G, Nuttal AL. Capsaicin stimulation of the cochlea and electrical stimulation of the trigeminal ganglion mediate vascular permeability in cochlear and vertebro-basilar arteries: a potential cause of inner ear dysfunction in headache. Neuroscience. 2001;103:189–201.

61. Goadsby PJ. The vascular theory of migraine–a great story wrecked by the facts. Brain. 2008;132:6–7.
62. Asghar MS, Hansen AE, Amin FM, et al. Evidence for a vascular factor in migraine. Ann Neurol. 2011;69:635–45.
63. Sauro KM, Becker WJ. The stress and migraine interaction. Headache J Head Face Pain. 2009;49:1378–86.
64. Stankewitz A, Aderjan D, Eippert F, May A. Trigeminal nociceptive transmission in migraineurs predicts migraine attacks. J Neurosci. 2011;31:1937–43.
65. Alstadhaug KB. Migraine and the hypothalamus. Cephalalgia. 2009;29:809–17.
66. Denuelle M, Fabre N, Payoux P, Chollet F, Geraud G. Hypothalamic activation in spontaneous migraine attacks. Headache J Head Face Pain. 2007;47: 1418–26.
67. Stankewitz A, May A. Increased limbic brainstem activity during migraine attacks following olfactory. Neurology. 2011;77:476–82.
68. Mainero C, Boshyan J, Hadjikhani N. Altered functional magnetic resonance imaging resting-state connectivity in periaqueductal gray networks in migraine. Ann Neurol. 2011;70:838–45.
69. Balaban CD, Ogburn SW, Warshafsky SG, Ahmed A, Yates BJ. Identification of neural networks that contribute to motion sickness through principal components analysis of Fos labeling induced by galvanic vestibular stimulation. PLoS One. 2014;9:e86730.

Vestibular Migraine in Childhood

4

Sharon L. Cushing

4.1 Introduction

The prevalence of vestibular and balance disorders in children is frequently underestimated. The reported frequency of these disorders ranges anywhere from 0.7 to 15 % [1–8]. While there is overlap between the differential diagnosis of vertigo presenting in adults and children, there are some etiologies found only in children. Such is the case of benign paroxysmal vertigo of childhood (BPVC) also known as benign recurrent vertigo of childhood (BRVC), a migraine variant. The prevalence, clinical presentation, natural history, and treatment of BPVC will be outlined in this chapter followed by a brief description of associated disorders and diagnoses with which BPVC is often confused.

S.L. Cushing, MD, MSc, FRCSC
Department of Otolaryngology Head and Neck Surgery, The Hospital for Sick Children, University of Toronto, 555 University Avenue, Room 6103C Burton Wing, Toronto, ON M5G 1X8, Canada

Archie's Cochlear Implant Laboratory, The Hospital for Sick Children, Toronto, ON, Canada
e-mail: sharon.cushing@sickkids.ca

4.2 Prevalence

In children with normal otoscopic findings, vertigo is commonly caused by migraine and migraine equivalents such as BPVC. In various reported cohorts of children presenting with vertigo, BPVC figures among the most common diagnoses, particularly in the young child, with prevalence ranging from 6 to 20 %. In the majority of these series, migrainous vertigo is reported separately from BPVC and represents a similar proportion of children presenting with vertigo [9–13].

4.3 Clinical Presentation

BPVC was initially described by Basser in 1964 [14]. This early description did not highlight an association with migraine, and it was in 1967 that Fenichel [15] first suggested a connection between childhood vertigo and migraine headache and coined the term "benign paroxysmal vertigo of childhood." This astute observation was based on the presence of a positive family history as well as the fact that, in some cases, the attacks changed from isolated vertigo to fairly typical migraine with time [15].

The diagnostic criteria for BPVC are outlined in section 1.3.3 in the International Classification of Headaches under the umbrella of "Childhood periodic syndromes that are common precursors of migraine" (Table 4.1) [16]. Specifically, BPVC is characterized by episodic vertigo that has a

S. Wetmore, A. Rubin (eds.), *Vestibular Migraine*,
DOI 10.1007/978-3-319-14550-1_4, © Springer International Publishing Switzerland 2015

Table 4.1 Description and diagnostic criteria for the diagnosis of benign paroxysmal vertigo of childhood according to the International Classification of Headaches, Childhood periodic syndromes that are common precursors of migraine, section 1.3.3 [16]

Description

This probably heterogeneous disorder is characterized by recurrent brief episodic attacks of vertigo occurring without warning and resolving spontaneously in otherwise healthy children

Diagnostic criteria

A. At least 5 attacks fulfilling criterion B

B. Multiple episodes of severe vertigo, occurring without warning and resolving spontaneously after minutes to hours

C. Normal neurological examination; audiometric and vestibular functions between attacks

D. Normal electroencephalogram

Note

Often associated with nystagmus or vomiting; unilateral throbbing headache may occur in some attacks

sudden onset and lasts from a few seconds to several minutes. The attack is not induced by movements of the head or specific positioning, differentiating it from benign paroxysmal positional vertigo (BPPV), with which it is often confused. Nausea, with or without vomiting, may be an associated symptom. Some children will articulate the sensation of spinning or describe the illusion of movement (i.e., "the house is shaking"). Typically, the child is frightened and seeks the support of adjacent objects (typically a parent) attempting not to fall. The postural instability can be so severe that it may cause the child to be limp and unable to remain upright without support. Abnormal eye movements suggestive of nystagmus may be seen, although this can be challenging as children will often shut their eyes during an acute attack. Parents, therefore, need to be instructed to specifically look for nystagmus. Furthermore, children are particularly good at suppressing nystagmus through fixation. It is likely for these reasons that nystagmus is observed and reported by a minority of parents.

A diagnosis of BPVC is one of exclusion, and, therefore, the most important characteristic is the absence of signs and symptoms that suggest another cause. With this in mind, the child does not experience any associated alterations of

consciousness, neurological changes, headache, or cochlear symptoms during the entire attack. The child also demonstrates a complete, and typically rapid, recovery with return to normal function.

A family history of migraine is both contributory and common in the child with BPVC with reports suggesting that this finding can be as high as 43 % [17]. As in migraine, children with BPVC will often report a history of motion intolerance most frequently manifested as "car sickness." In recent literature, there is a suggestion that creatine kinase levels are elevated in BPVC and its measurement may help in the diagnosis [18]. However, this has not become standard clinical practice. Given the overlap in the clinical presentation between BPVC and epileptic vertigo, EEG is often added to a complete neurologic exam and should be normal in the setting of BPVC.

The age of onset of BPVC is variable and reports in the literature range from 18 months to 12 years. However, it most frequently occurs prior to 4 years of age and is uncommon after 8 years [14]. On average, the episodes may occur every 4–6 weeks, with the intervals ranging from once a week to every 6 months. Typically, the frequency of attacks decreases with age. Similar to migraine, BPVC has a higher prevalence in females [19].

4.4 Pathophysiology

The pathophysiology of BPVC is as yet unproven; however, there is presumed overlap with the underlying pathophysiology for migraine. More specifically, vertigo in the setting of migraine is theorized to result from vascular alterations that produce a transient hypoxia of the vestibular nuclei and the vestibular pathways [20].

4.5 Peripheral Vestibular Testing in BPVC

While the original report by Basser suggested peripheral vestibular dysfunction based on findings of moderate to complete canal paresis in response to a caloric stimulus, evidence of peripheral dysfunction in the setting of BPVC has not been found by others [13, 21, 22]. As a result, in the presence of a history consistent with BPVC and a normal, complete neuro-otologic exam, ancillary vestibular end-organ testing (e.g., horizontal canal response to caloric or rotational testing and saccular response by vestibular evoked myogenic testing) may not be necessary at the outset. If additional symptoms evolve or if the pattern of episodes differs from the expected natural history of BPVC, peripheral vestibular testing should be considered. Despite the absence of peripheral vestibular loss, a subtle delay in gross motor development has been noted [21]. In addition, some reports suggest that behavioral difficulties, anxiety, depressive, and hyperactivity symptoms are more common in children with BPVC [23].

4.6 Diagnostic Imaging

Most clinicians would suggest that imaging (typically magnetic resonance imaging (MRI)) is unnecessary in the presence of a convincing history for BPVC. The challenge in managing these children is that families often remain concerned about serious central nervous system causes, such as a brain tumor. It is often difficult to reassure them definitively in the absence of confirmatory imaging. Our experience is that frequently these children will have already undergone imaging ordered by their primary care physician prior to being seen in consultation. If the vertigo does not improve on an expected timeline or additional symptoms evolve, MRI should be considered to exclude a central cause.

4.7 Natural History

Beyond making the diagnosis, the role of the clinician is to inform and reassure parents of the benign nature of this condition that in most cases does not require specific treatment. BPVC has a favorable outlook, and long-term follow-up studies have shown complete resolution along a variety of timelines [24]. A history of BPVC is associated with an increased risk of developing more classic migraine later on in life. In the

literature, risk estimates range from 13 to 21 %. These estimates include the development of both classic migraine and other associated symptoms such as cyclic vomiting, recurrent abdominal pain, scotomata, and photophobia [17, 24].

4.8 Treatment

As outlined above, the primary treatment of BPVC primarily relates to reassuring the family of the benign, self-limiting nature of the disease. Once this is understood, most families are happy to cope with the individual episodes and do not request any additional treatment. Beyond reassurance, a conservative treatment, if deemed necessary, would include eliminating factors that trigger a crisis, similar to migraine. Parents may be able to identify such triggers including poor or irregular sleep, intake of certain foods, and stress. In the uncommon situation where attacks are frequent and disabling, a pharmacological approach can be entertained. In children, this typically begins with magnesium replacement followed by prophylactic medications, in keeping with the pharmacological management of more classic migraine. Vestibular suppressants and abortive migraine medications are not helpful in the setting of BPVC because of the short duration of symptoms. In general, the threshold for pharmacological treatment in children is higher than in adults, and in the setting of BPVC, most clinicians find pharmacological treatment unnecessary. If the attacks of vertigo are so severe or frequent to warrant pharmacologic treatment, the clinician may wish to reconsider the diagnosis of BPVC and expand the diagnostic work-up.

4.9 Associated Conditions

Included in section 1.3.3 in the International Classification of Headaches under the umbrella of "Childhood periodic syndromes that are common precursors of migraine" is abdominal migraine. This condition is characterized by recurrent episodic attacks of vomiting, intense nausea associated with pallor and lethargy, as well as midline, moderate to severe intensity abdominal pain. These attacks last 1–72 h with normality between episodes [16].

In addition to abdominal migraine, although not formally defined in the International Classification of Headaches, many authors suggest that benign paroxysmal torticollis of infancy is a migraine-related disorder [25, 26]. It is clinically characterized as a self-limiting condition, in which the child typically wakes in the morning with direction-varying head tilt lasting anywhere from a few hours to many days, with nighttime relief. Symptoms present typically within the first few months of life and resolve by age 3–4 years. Recently, paroxysmal torticollis, like BPVC, has been associated with gross and fine motor delay [27]. Children with abdominal migraine or benign paroxysmal torticollis of infancy may go on to develop BPVC and/or more classic migraine.

4.10   Other Diagnoses in the Differential

While there is a lengthy differential for the presentation of vertigo in children, those diagnoses that mimic BPVC are few. The following discussion will be limited to those conditions that are most frequently confused with BPVC.

Vertigo that lasts seconds to minutes can be attributed not only to benign paroxysmal vertigo of childhood (BPVC) but also to benign paroxysmal positional vertigo (BPPV). While similar in name (and acronym), these two entities are very different but often confused. While the majority of clinicians are familiar with BPPV, many have never heard of the entity of BPVC. As a result, many children with BPVC are misdiagnosed with BPPV. While BPPV is one of the most common causes of vertigo in adults, it is very uncommon in children. The exception to this rule is the child who presents with BPPV after having suffered a concussion or subsequent to surgical intervention such as cochlear implantation. The main differentiating factor is that BPPV occurs repeatedly in response to specific head position. This can be difficult to tease out in

young children who often find themselves through play in a variety of head-hanging positions, thus blurring the distinction between BPVC and BPPV further.

It is important also to distinguish BPVC from a seizure disorder because these children can present in a very similar fashion. Epileptic vertigo is a rare type of focal seizure due to epileptic activity arising from parts of the brain that represent the vestibular system, including the frontal, temporal, and parietal cortex. Vertigo resulting from epilepsy can present in clusters of very brief episodes (seconds to minutes) therefore mimicking the time course of BPVC. When the vertiginous symptoms are accompanied by confusion, focal sensory, or motor symptoms, or a convulsion, the diagnosis of epilepsy becomes more obvious although, in many instances, these associated symptoms are absent or subtle. Epileptic vertigo can be associated with a loss of consciousness although this may not accompany every episode. Many children may have difficulty articulating focal sensory or motor symptoms making differentiation of BPVC from epilepsy exceedingly difficult. Thankfully, isolated vertigo as a sole manifestation of a seizure is very rare, and ultimately, symptoms and signs will evolve into recognition. In any child presenting with vertigo where seizure figures into the differential, the threshold for ordering an EEG should be low. In the setting of epileptic vertigo, temporal paroxysmal discharges or diffuse paroxysmal discharges are most frequently seen on the EEG [28]. It is however important to remember that a single normal EEG study does not rule out the possibility of seizures; when the index of suspicion for seizure is high, extended, video, or sleep-deprived EEG may be warranted. Therefore, when considering a diagnosis of BPVC, one should always consider and be mindful of even the most subtle signs of epileptic vertigo.

4.11   Summary

A variety of peripheral vestibular causes can lead to vertigo and disequilibrium in the pediatric population. The underlying etiologic distribution is considerably different than the adult population, and, in general, children compensate much more rapidly to acute changes in vestibular function. The biggest risk factors for the development of peripheral vestibular dysfunction in children include an associated SNHL and head trauma. The most common form of vertigo in a young child with an otherwise normal otoscopic exam is BPVC, a migraine variant. A thorough and age-appropriate evaluation of both balance and vestibular end-organ function should be performed in children presenting with such complaints. Once familiar with its clinical presentation, as well as that of the other conditions with which it is often confused, a diagnosis of BPVC is one that can be easily recognized in the clinic.

References

1. O'Reilly RC, Morlet T, Nicholas BD, Josephson G, Horlbeck D, Lundy L, et al. Prevalence of vestibular and balance disorders in children. Otol Neurotol. 2010;31(9):1441–4.
2. Worden BF, Blevins NH. Pediatric vestibulopathy and pseudovestibulopathy: differential diagnosis and management. Curr Opin Otolaryngol Head Neck Surg. 2007;15(5):304–9.
3. Eviatar L, Bergtraum M, Randel RM. Post-traumatic vertigo in children: a diagnostic approach. Pediatr Neurol. 1986;2(2):61–6.
4. Riina N, Ilmari P, Kentala E. Vertigo and imbalance in children: a retrospective study in a Helsinki University otorhinolaryngology clinic. Arch Otolaryngol Head Neck Surg. 2005;131(11):996–1000.
5. Niemensivu R, Pyykko I, Wiener-Vacher SR, Kentala E. Vertigo and balance problems in children– an epidemiologic study in Finland. Int J Pediatr Otorhinolaryngol. 2006;70(2):259–65.
6. Abu-Arafeh I, Russell G. Paroxysmal vertigo as a migraine equivalent in children: a population-based study. Cephalalgia. 1995;15(1):22–5; discussion 4.
7. Russell G, Abu-Arafeh I. Paroxysmal vertigo in children–an epidemiological study. Int J Pediatr Otorhinolaryngol. 1999;49 Suppl 1:S105–7.
8. Bower CM, Cotton RT. The spectrum of vertigo in children. Arch Otolaryngol Head Neck Surg. 1995;121(8):911–5.
9. Choung YH, Park K, Moon SK, Kim CH, Ryu SJ. Various causes and clinical characteristics in vertigo in children with normal eardrums. Int J Pediatr Otorhinolaryngol. 2003;67(8):889–94.
10. Erbek SH, Erbek SS, Yilmaz I, Topal O, Ozgirgin N, Ozluoglu LN, et al. Vertigo in childhood: a clinical experience. Int J Pediatr Otorhinolaryngol. 2006;70(9):1547–54.
11. McCaslin DL, Jacobson GP, Gruenwald JM. The predominant forms of vertigo in children and their associated findings on balance function testing. Otolaryngol Clin North Am. 2011;44(2):291–307, vii.
12. Wiener-Vacher SR. Vestibular disorders in children. Int J Audiol. 2008;47(9):578–83.
13. Weisleder P, Fife TD. Dizziness and headache: a common association in children and adolescents. J Child Neurol. 2001;16(10):727–30.
14. Basser LS. Benign paroxysmal vertigo of childhood. (A variety of vestibular neuronitis). Brain J Neurol. 1964;87:141–52.
15. Fenichel GM. Migraine as a cause of benign paroxysmal vertigo of childhood. J Pediatr. 1967;71(1):114–5.
16. Society SotIH. The international classification of headache disorders. Cephalalgia. 2004;24 (Suppl 1):9–160. 2nd edition.
17. Parker C. Complicated migraine syndromes and migraine variants. Pediatr Ann. 1997;26(7):417–21.
18. Rodoo P, Hellberg D. Creatine kinase MB (CK-MB) in benign paroxysmal vertigo of childhood: a new diagnostic marker. J Pediatr. 2005;146(4):548–51.
19. Al-Twaijri WA, Shevell MI. Pediatric migraine equivalents: occurrence and clinical features in practice. Pediatr Neurol. 2002;26(5):365–8.
20. Perez Plasencia D, Beltran Mateos LD, del Canizo Alvarez A, Sancipriano JA, Calvo Boizas E, Benito Gonzalez JJ. Benign paroxysmal vertigo in childhood. Acta Otorrinolaringol Esp. 1998;49(2):151–5.
21. O'Reilly RC, Greywoode J, Morlet T, Miller F, Henley J, Church C, et al. Comprehensive vestibular and balance testing in the dizzy pediatric population. Otolaryngol Head Neck Surg. 2011;144(2):142–8.
22. Mira E, Piacentino G, Lanzi G, Balottin U. Benign paroxysmal vertigo in childhood. Diagnostic significance of vestibular examination and headache provocation tests. Acta Otolaryngol. 1984;406:271–4.
23. Reale L, Guarnera M, Grillo C, Maiolino L, Ruta L, Mazzone L. Psychological assessment in children and adolescents with benign paroxysmal vertigo. Brain Dev. 2011;33(2):125–30.
24. Lindskog U, Odkvist L, Noaksson L, Wallquist J. Benign paroxysmal vertigo in childhood: a long-term follow-up. Headache. 1999;39(1):33–7.
25. Deonna T, Martin D. Benign paroxysmal torticollis in infancy. Arch Dis Child. 1981;56(12):956–9.
26. Drigo P, Carli G, Laverda AM. Benign paroxysmal torticollis of infancy. Brain Dev. 2000;22(3):169–72.
27. Rosman NP, Douglass LM, Sharif UM, Paolini J. The neurology of benign paroxysmal torticollis of infancy: report of 10 new cases and review of the literature. J Child Neurol. 2009;24(2):155–60.
28. Eviatar L, Eviatar A. Vertigo in children: differential diagnosis and treatment. Pediatrics. 1977;59(6):833–8.

Treatment of Vestibular Migraine

5

Adam M. Cassis and Yuri Agrawal

5.1 Introduction

The symptoms of migrainous headache and dizziness are quite common and often are related to each other. Studies have shown that patients with migraine are three times more likely to have experienced dizziness than controls [1, 2]. In patients presenting with vertigo, 30–50 % of those patients have or previously had a diagnosis of migraine [3, 4]. Population-based studies have shown a prevalence of migraine of 17 % in women and 6 % in men, while dizziness is experienced by 20 % of the general population [5, 6]. Comparing a group of patients from a dizzy clinic showed the diagnosis of migraine was higher than in the control group (age- and sex-matched orthopedic patients), 38 % versus 24 % [7].

The pathophysiology of VM is not fully understood. The common absence of a temporal connection between headaches and vestibular symptoms make it difficult to link traditional migraine pathophysiology and VM. Thus, targeting pharmacologic treatment for these patients can be difficult. A phenomenon known as cortical spreading depression (CSD) that has been observed in migraine patients is thought to be responsible for the aura symptoms. This process may also account for some of the vestibular symptoms experienced by patients [8–13].

5.2 Treatment of Vestibular Migraine

Treatment of VM should be tailored to each individual patient. For some patients, attacks of dizziness are mild and infrequent; VM does not cause a disturbance in their daily lives. However, some patients have severe, frequent, or prolonged attacks that necessitate intervention.

5.2.1 Treatment: General Concepts

While the mainstay to treating VM is pharmacotherapy, treatments other than medications have been used with success. These consist largely of dietary modifications, lifestyle changes, and vestibular physical therapy. Strategies to treat vestibular migraine are often modeled after similar strategies to treat migraine headaches. Similar to Menière's disease, patients may notice triggers

A.M. Cassis, MD (✉)
Department of Otolaryngology,
West Virginia University Hospital,
HSC, P.O. Box 9200, Morgantown,
WV 26506, USA
e-mail: acassis1@hsc.wvu.edu

Y. Agrawal, MD
Department of Otolaryngology-Head and Neck
Surgery, Johns Hopkins,
601 North Caroline Street, 6th Floor Outpatient
Center, Baltimore, MD 21287, USA
e-mail: yagrawa1@jhmi.edu

S. Wetmore, A. Rubin (eds.), *Vestibular Migraine*,
DOI 10.1007/978-3-319-14550-1_5, © Springer International Publishing Switzerland 2015

that bring on an episode of migraine. These include certain foods, stress, sleep disturbance, or hormonal changes such as menses/menopause. Studies have shown that dietary modification (avoidance of caffeine, alcohol, aged wines and cheeses, chocolate, and artificial sweeteners such as aspartame) has been effective in controlling symptoms [14, 15]. Avoidance of these triggers is a noninvasive and an easy "first step" in treating VM and may be better accepted initially than pharmacologic intervention.

Medications to treat VM are the same medications that are used to treat migraine headaches. These consist of abortive and prophylactic medications. The current quality of the literature to support pharmacologic treatment of VM is modest. Although some studies have looked particularly at vestibular migraine, many report on the treatment of migraine aura, which may or may not consist of vestibular symptoms. Only recently have specific diagnostic criteria for VM been established [7, 16]. The most current diagnostic criteria were released in a joint document from the Barany Society and the Migraine Classification Subcommittee of the International Headache Society [17]. A more detailed discussion of the diagnostic criteria is reviewed in Chap. 2. Despite the diagnostic criteria, there is still nonuniformity with which the data is collected, analyzed, and reported. In addition, there have been no randomized, placebo-controlled trials to evaluate the efficacy of prophylactic migraine medications for VM. We must therefore rely on retrospective reviews and case reports to judge the usefulness of prophylactic medications.

5.2.2 Abortive Medications

Several studies have evaluated the efficacy of abortive migraine medications for the treatment of VM. The only randomized, double-blinded, placebo-controlled drug trial for the treatment of VM was a study performed by Neuhauser and colleagues [18]. The drug zolmitriptan was used as an abortive agent in patients who met criteria for VM. The response rate of the vestibular symptoms to zolmitriptan was 38 %, while the

placebo garnered a 22 % response. Due to a significant lack of power in this study, these results were inconclusive. A study performed by Bikhazi et al. looked at the efficacy of prophylactic versus abortive migraine agents (specifically sumatriptan) for alleviating symptoms of headache and vestibular symptoms. They found that patients treated with sumatriptan had a better response of their vestibular and headache symptoms than did the group treated with prophylactic medications. Also in the same study, they found that the group of abortive agents (ergots, NSAIDs, opiates, and sumatriptan) was helpful in relieving vestibular and headache symptoms [19].

There are scattered reports of medications being used to abort prolonged migraine aura symptoms, although none specifically mention an aura consisting of vestibular symptoms. Prakash treated four patients who presented with prolonged symptoms with intravenous methylprednisone, and they responded well to treatment [20]. Furosemide and acetazolamide have also been used to abort migraine aura status in two case series, although there was no mention that the aura included vestibular symptoms [21, 22]. Abortive medications may be useful for those patients who have prolonged symptoms, especially for those with coexistent headaches.

Some patients with VM have short spells of dizziness lasting from seconds to minutes, while others have constant lingering symptoms, making abortive medications difficult to use. Prophylactic medications make more sense for these patients. The bulk of the literature on treatment of vestibular migraine is focused on prophylactic medical therapy. Medications prescribed for VM prophylaxis are drugs historically used to prevent migraine headaches.

5.2.3 Prophylactic Medications

Migraine prophylactic medications are usually in one of three categories: antihypertensives (beta-blockers, calcium channel blockers), antidepressives (tricyclic antidepressants, SSRIs, and SNRIs), or neuroleptic medications (topiramate, gabapentin, lamotrigine, valproate, benzodiazepines). There are reports of success in treating migraine with various other medications, such as acetazolamide, furosemide, and corticosteroids. These different medication classes act on different pathophysiologic pathways to mitigate the symptoms of migraine. For an extensive review of migraine pathophysiology and mechanism of action of migraine prophylactic drugs, please review articles by Buchanan and Ramadan [6, 23].

Beta-blockers (BBs) act by preventing central hypersensitivity by inhibiting norepinephrine release, antagonizing 5-HT receptors, inhibiting nitric oxide (NO) synthase, as well as acting synergistically with N-methyl-D-aspartate (NMDA) blockers [6]. Commonly used medications in this class include propranolol and metoprolol. These medications are useful for treating patients with preexisting hypertension, essential tremor, panic attacks, or anxiety. This class of medication should be avoided in patient with diabetes mellitus or depression and is contraindicated in those with congestive heart failure, Raynaud's disease, and asthma.

Calcium channel blockers (CCBs) are also another popular antihypertensive class of drugs that have been used for treatment of VM. They act to inhibit a migraine headache by blocking voltage-gated calcium channels that may modulate neuronal activity. Also, blockage of calcium channels on calcitonin gene-related peptide (CGRP) neurons inhibits CGRP release, which is an important step in the inflammatory cascade in migraine pathology. Verapamil and flunarizine (not marketed in the United States) are commonly used medications in this class. CCBs work as well for patients with hypertension, especially those with lung conditions such as asthma. They are contraindicated in those patients with cardiac conduction abnormalities. Constipation is the most common side effect.

Tricyclic antidepressants (TCAs) are another common class of medications used in the treatment of VM. TCAs have long been used in the treatment of migraine and chronic pain. Their mechanism of action consists of enhancement of antinociceptive neurons, downregulation of 5-hydroxytryptamine (HT2) receptors, blockage of sodium channels (thereby modulating peripheral sensitization), and increase in gamma-aminobutyric acid (GABA) levels. Often this medication is chosen when patients have comorbid conditions such as depression and chronic tension headaches. Caution must be exercised with patients with epilepsy and those with cardiac arrhythmias (may cause QT interval prolongation). Sexual dysfunction, weight gain, sedation, and orthostatic hypotension are common side effects.

Neuroleptic medications have been well studied in migraine. The most studied drugs are sodium valproate, topiramate, and lamotrigine. Valproate increases presynaptic levels of GABA, thereby increasing overall GABA activity. Valproate also inhibits the enzymatic degradation of GABA. Weight gain and hair loss can be experienced with this medication. Routine monitoring is required when prescribing this medication due to its risk of pancreatitis and hepatotoxicity and therefore should not be used in patients with liver disease. Lamotrigine acts by inhibiting glutamate secretion (a neurotransmitter associated with CSD), while topiramate potentiates GABA activity and blocks calcium channels. Both lamotrigine and topiramate block voltage-sensitive sodium channels, which may play a role in vestibular migraine pathogenesis. Topiramate is also an inhibitor of carbonic anhydrase activity, similar to that of acetazolamide. Common side effects of topiramate include dizziness, somnolence, and weight loss. Lamotrigine has similar side effects, but rare adverse reactions to this medication include serious rash (Stevens-Johnson syndrome, toxic epidermal necrolysis), hypersensitivity, multi-organ failure, and blood dyscrasias.

Generally speaking, prophylactic medications are started at a low dose and increased as needed for control of symptoms or tolerability. Often, multiple medications may need to be tried, alone or in combination, to achieve symptom control [15, 24]. While first-line medications may be chosen based on physician preference and/or familiarity, others are used in either a stepwise fashion or tailored to the individual patient based on their medical history. Table 5.1 shows reported doses of various drugs used in the literature.

Table 5.1 Prescribed doses as described in the literature

Drug	Median dose (mg/day)	Range (mg/day)
Topiramate	50	25–125
Valproic Acid	600	300–800
Lamotrigine	75	50–150
Propranolol	160	40–240
Metoprolol	150	50–250
Amitriptyline	50	10–100
Nortriptyline	50	10–75
Sertraline	50	–
Fluoxetine	–	20–40
Clonazepam	1.0	0.125–2.0
Alpreazolam	–	0.125–0.25
Lorazepam	–	1.0–1.5
Prazepam	30	–
Butterbur root	50	50–150

Of the above-listed medications, only topiramate, valproic acid, and propranolol are FDA approved for the treatment of migraine headache. There are no medications currently FDA approved for VM

5.2.4 Review of the Literature

In a retrospective review of 19 patients, Bisdorff evaluated the efficacy of lamotrigine in treating patients with migraine headaches with vertigo. The dose was 100 mg/day and the patients were followed for 3–4 months. At the end of the observational period, the frequency of vertigo attacks was significantly decreased. Vertigo duration and headache frequency were also reduced, although not to a statistically significant extent. This medication was well tolerated in this group of patients [25].

Other studies evaluating the effect of lamotrigine on migraine aura found it to be quite effective, although no study specifically mentioned vestibular migraine. An animal study evaluating CSD in rats showed that lamotrigine was effective in reducing CSD, while valproate and riboflavin had no effect [9]. Lampl and colleagues conducted an open longitudinal pilot study of lamotrigine on 15 patients who had migraine with aura. Dosing was started at 25 mg a day. The dose was titrated up as needed to a maximum dose of 100 mg/day to control the patient's symptoms. All patients responded favorably to the medication with a decreased frequency and severity of their aura symptoms [10]. A small case series showed lamotrigine to be effective in basilar migraine with aura, although no specific reference to vestibular symptoms was made [26]. Other studies have shown an overall decrease in aura frequency, with one study showing resolution of a prolonged aura (months to years) after treatment with lamotrigine [11–13].

Although valproate has been well studied for migraine headache prophylaxis, only one study has investigated its effects on VM. Celiker et al. studied the effects of valproic acid on three groups of migraine patients: migraine with vertigo, migraine with dizziness, and migraine without vestibular symptoms. They also compared electronystagmographic findings between the groups, both before and after treatment. Two of the original 43 patients dropped out due to medication side effects. There was a significant decrease in the number of attacks in the migraine with vertigo and the migraine with dizziness group ($p < 0.001$). There was also a significant decrease in vestibular symptoms in patients whose symptoms were not related to the headache period. ENG findings did not change between the pretreatment and post-treatment conditions [27].

There have been two studies investigating topiramate as a prophylactic treatment of VM. The first consisted of a group of 10 patients who met the Neuhauser criteria. The average dose patients received was 100 mg/day. One of those patients stopped taking the medication due to side effects. The other 9 patients were without vestibular symptoms at the end of a 9-month period, with only 2 of those patients experiencing an attack over that time frame [28]. The second was an open-label study looking at the effect of topiramate at different doses, 50 and 100 mg/day. Fifteen patients were recruited into both groups. Both efficacy and tolerability were studied. In the low-dose group, 14 of 15 patients had improvement of their vertigo symptoms, with 6 of those having complete relief of their symptoms and only 1 having no change. All patients tolerated this dose well. In the high-dose group, 12 of 15 had improvement in their dizzy symptoms, while 3 had no change. Four patients in this group could not tolerate the high dose and dropped out in the first month of the study. Overall there was no difference between the two dosing groups in regard to vertigo severity and frequency [29]. In a study by Lampl looking at migraine aura and topiramate, the authors found that the drug improved headache symptoms, although did not statistically influence aura frequency or duration [30].

Similar to other migraine prophylactic medications, levetiracetam (an antiseizure medication) has inhibitory effects on neuronal calcium channels. An open-label trial consisting of 16 patients with migraine with aura were treated with levetiracetam for 6 months at a dose of 1,000 mg/day. The frequency of attacks was significantly reduced over the first month ($p < 0.001$). Attack frequency was further reduced in the second month ($p < 0.001$) and again in the third month ($p < 0.001$). This effect persisted over the next 3 months. Duration of the aura was decreased as well. Six of these patients had minor side effects (dizziness, nervousness, somnolence), but none stopped taking the medication [31].

There have been a handful of studies that compared various different prophylactic medications within one study. These medications were prescribed according to a specific treatment algorithm or in a nonstandardized fashion according to specific patient characteristics. In a series of 100 patients, Baier et al. reviewed their series of patients treated for VM. Of the 100 patients, 74 were prescribed prophylactic medications for their symptoms. These were delivered in a nonstandardized fashion. The remaining 26 patients were treated with conservative therapy consisting of dietary modifications, lifestyle changes, physical therapy, and progressive muscle relaxation. All patients treated pharmacologically showed a decrease in vertigo duration, intensity, and frequency. The conservative therapy group only showed a decrease in vertigo intensity. Of the patients treated with pharmacologic therapy, five stopped the medications due to side effects (4 beta-blocker, 1 calcium channel blocker) [32].

Another large series of 89 patients compared outcomes for treatment of VM. Of the 89 patients, 59 (66 %) were treated with dietary changes, 7 % were treated with lifestyle changes, and balance physical therapy is used in 27 %. Prophylactic medications were used in 79 of those 89 patients, and the initial drug of choice was tailored to the specific patient based on the medical history. Benzodiazepines were the most commonly prescribed medication, alone or in combination, at 90 % (clonazepam most often). TCAs were used in 42 % of patients, and beta-blockers were used in 33 % of patients. SSRIs and calcium channel blockers were used, but to a lesser degree. In this series of patients, 44 % of patients only needed a single medication, with 33 % requiring two medications, either alone or in combination. Likewise, 15 % used three medications, with the rest using four or more medications (again, alone or in combination) to achieve symptom control. At the time of symptom control, 67 % required only one medication and 25 % needed two medications, with the rest of the patients requiring three or more medications for symptom control. All 10 patients treated with non-pharmacologic measures were continuing this treatment at follow-up. Out of the 79 patients treated with medications, 60 were still taking their medications. Of the 19 that stopped the medication, 8 stopped due to symptom control, 7 had symptoms under satisfactory control, 3 had significant side effects, and 1 stopped due to lack of control of symptoms. Of the patients with episodic vertigo, 92 % had either a complete response or had significant improvement in their symptoms. This same degree of improvement was achieved in 89 % of patients with positional vertigo and 86 % with non-vertiginous dizziness. Although the majority of patients were treated with medications, outcomes were not reported in regard to medical therapy versus dietary/lifestyle modification or a combination thereof [15].

Maione reported on his series of 53 patients with VM. Again, medications were chosen in a nonrandomized fashion based on the patient's characteristics, drug properties, and side effects. The most common medications used were beta-blockers, benzodiazepines, and calcium channel blockers, in that order. Eight patients needed to have their medication changed due to side effects, inefficacy, or a contraindication based on a new diagnosis. Some females underwent estrogenic management as well (2 patients). No mention of dietary or lifestyles changes was made. The outcomes in these patients were as follows: 28 % had complete control of symptoms, 42 % had substantial control, 20 % moderate control, and 11 % had minimal or no control of their symptoms. Of those with recurrent vertigo spells, complete resolution of their spells occurred in 58 %, a >50 % reduction of attacks in 24 %, <50 % reduction of attacks in 15 %, and no reduction in 3 % [24].

Alternatively, some centers base therapy on a treatment algorithm. In a series of 81 patients, Reploeg and Goebel treated patients in a stepwise fashion. First-line treatment was dietary modification. If symptoms were not controlled on dietary modification alone, patients were started on 10 or 25 mg of nortriptyline and titrated up to 50 mg for symptom control. If this did not result in symptom control, atenolol was prescribed at 25 mg and was titrated up to 50 mg if necessary, usually as monotherapy, but occasionally atenolol was used in addition to nortriptyline. For symptoms that persisted beyond this, a neurology consultation was obtained. Overall, 72 % had complete or greater than 75 % reduction of the frequency of their symptoms. Thirteen of the 81 patients responded to dietary modifications alone. Those who needed nortriptyline along with dietary modifications had an overall 78 % response rate to this treatment. The response rate of diet plus beta-blocker/other drugs (SSRI, CCB, valproic acid, carbamazepine, and gabapentin) was 57 %. Of those prescribed nortriptyline, 3 of 68 could not tolerate the medication due to side effects, with 1 of 19 stopping their beta-blocker for the same reason [14].

A similar approach was used by Mikulec and colleagues. In patients with VM, a caffeine cessation trial was instituted for the first 4–6 weeks of treatment. They were then assigned to receive nortriptyline or topiramate. Of those patients who did not respond favorably to the medication, some were switched with the other study drug (i.e., nortriptyline nonresponders were prescribed topiramate and vice versa). Five out of the 34 (15 %) patients treated with caffeine restriction alone had some response to reduction in their caffeine intake, although all went on to be treated with medications. The response in patients receiving nortriptyline was 57 %, while the response rate for topiramate as 17 %. Overall success rate for diet modification with or without medications was 75 % [33].

In 2005, Furman and colleagues proposed a new disorder, migraine-anxiety-related dizziness, or MARD, citing overlap between migraine, anxiety, and balance disorders as well as a high incidence of psychiatric comorbidities in patients with migraine. In this population of patients where vestibular symptoms predominated, prophylactic therapy with an antidepressant (imipramine/sertraline) plus benzodiazepine (clonazepam/diazepam) was recommended. In those patients where anxiety predominated, an SSRI such as paroxetine was recommended; benzodiazepines were used as a supplementary medication for those with significant anxiety and balance symptoms [34].

Acetazolamide has been shown to be useful in treating familial hemiplegic migraine with essential tremor. Baloh published a series of five patients, all from the same family, who had a reduction in their vertigo spells in addition to decreased severity of migraine headaches and tremor [35].

Physical therapy for vestibular symptoms of migraine seems to be effective. Several studies have demonstrated both peripheral and central vestibular abnormalities on ENG. Oculomotor and vestibulo-ocular reflex abnormalities are common in VM patients [36–38]. One study reviewed 14 patients with a diagnosis of VM who were treated with a customized physical therapy exercise program over a 4-month period. The treatment plans consisted of various components, including general strength and stretching exercises, habituation exercises, vestibular compensation exercises, balance and gait training, or enhancing the use of specific sensory inputs for balance control. Outcome measures used were pre-and posttreatment questionnaires using the Dizziness Handicap Inventory (DHI), Activities-Specific Balance Confidence Scale (ABC), and the Dynamic Gait Index (DGI). After the study period of 4 months was over, the

DHI improved by 12 points ($p < .01$), the ABC improved by 14 points ($p < .01$), and DGI improved by 4 points ($p < .01$). The number of falls also decreased by 78 % ($p < .05$), while baseline dizzy symptoms decreased significantly as well ($p < .05$) [39]. Another study looked at two groups of patients with vestibular symptoms (with or without a history of migraine) who also underwent a customized physical therapy program. The same outcome measures were used as in the previously mentioned study (DHI, ABC, DGI), as well as the Timed Up and Go Test. Both groups demonstrated improvements in both subjective and objective measures after physical therapy. Patients with migraine perceived a greater handicap than patients without migraine that was greater than the gap in physical performance between the two groups [40]. These findings were corroborated by another study that compared physical therapy outcomes for patients with vestibular symptoms with or without migraine. They also found that patients with VM had poorer performance at the onset of therapy compared to those without migraine. The degree of improvement was similar for both groups although the group of patients with VM on vestibular suppressants tended to do worse. Compliance was excellent in both groups [37].

A study of the long-term course of VM is useful for physicians and patients in understanding expected outcomes over time. In a longitudinal study, 61 patients with VM were followed over an average of 9 years. The majority (87 %) of these patients still reported vertigo attacks during that period. The remaining patients (13 %) had been vertigo-free for an average of 6.6 years. During that time span, 22 (36 %) patients had taken prophylaxis for their symptoms, but only 8 (13 %) were still taking their medication, 2 of which were in the vertigo-free group. Every patient still experienced migraine headaches, except for one. Overall vertigo frequency decreased in 56 %, increased in 29 %, and was unchanged in 16 %. Patients with cochlear symptoms related to the vertigo attacks increased from 16 to 49 % over the study period. On neurotologic testing, peripheral vestibular dysfunction or oculomotor dysfunction increased from 18 to 47.5 %, although patients with oculomotor dysfunction had variable test results over time with some patients reverting back to normal findings on later examination. Patients reported interictal dizziness related to motion sickness or self-motion in 69 %, visual-induced symptoms in 54 %, and a mild persistent dizziness in 18 % of patients. On caloric testing, the incidence of a unilateral canal paresis increased from 5 to 16 %. This study demonstrates the high incidence and persistence of symptoms in patients with VM and underscores the need for prophylactic medical therapy in this population [41].

Conclusion

VM is a common cause of dizziness and is thought to be the second most common cause of vertigo after BPPV. The current data on VM treatment is largely of poor quality. The literature still lacks a randomized, double-blind, placebo-controlled study for the treatment of VM. Only recently the Barany Society and the International Headache Society published a proposal concerning diagnostic criteria for vestibular migraine, but outcome measures for treatment are still nonstandardized, making comparisons difficult.

For those patients with minor or infrequent vestibular symptoms, a vestibular suppressant such as promethazine, meclizine, metoclopramide, or diazepam is a good option with the main side effect consisting of sedation; diazepam can also be habit forming. Abortive migraine medications such as sumatriptan or zolmitriptan may be useful as well, especially if headaches occur with the vestibular symptoms.

However, many patients have symptoms that do not lend themselves well to abortive treatment, those with dizziness lasting seconds to minutes or those with prolonged or constant daily symptoms. Non-pharmacologic management principles (dietary modification, regular sleep, stress reduction, physical therapy) can be useful in treating those patients with relatively minor or infrequent symptoms. For those patients who do not respond to conservative treatment, prophylaxis with drugs is warranted.

One can take many approaches to treating patients with prophylactic medical therapy for VM. Patients may be treated as part of a protocol and in a stepwise fashion. This usually consists of dietary and lifestyle modifications plus a migraine prophylactic medication with which the treating physician is familiar. Another approach is to prescribe medications based on the patient's characteristics, comorbidities, and side effects. With a wide array of medications to choose from, monotherapy and sometimes multidrug regimens are quite effective in relieving patient's symptoms.

References

1. Kuritzky A, Ziegler DK, Hassanein R. Vertigo, motion sickness and migraine. Headache. 1981;21(5):227–31.
2. Kayan A, Hood JD. Neuro-otological manifestations of migraine. Brain. 1984;107(Pt 4):1123–42.
3. Aragones JM, Fortes–Rego J, Fuste J, Cardozo A. Migraine: an alternative in the diagnosis of unclassified vertigo. Headache. 1993;33:125–8.
4. Savundra PA, Carroll JD, Davies RA, Luxon LM. Migraine associated vertigo. Cephalagia. 1997;17:505–10.
5. Kroenke K, Price RK. Symptoms in the community. Prevalence, classification, and psychiatric comorbidity. Arch Intern Med. 1993;153(21):2474–80.
6. Stewart WF, Simon D, Shechter A, Lipton RB. Population variation in migraine prevalence: a meta-analysis. J Clin Epidemiol. 1995;48:269–80.
7. Neuhauser H, Leopold M, von Brevern M, Arnold G, Lempert T. The interrelations of migraine, vertigo, and migrainous vertigo. Neurology. 2001;56(4):436–41.
8. Buchanan TM, Ramadan NM. Prophylactic pharmacotherapy for migraine headaches. Semin Neurol. 2006;26(2):188–98.
9. Bogdanov VB, Multon S, Chauvel V, Bogdanova OV, Prodanov D, Makarchuk MY, Schoenen J. Migraine preventive drugs differentially affect cortical spreading depression in rat. Neurobiol Dis. 2011;41(2):430–5.
10. Lampl C, Katsarava Z, Diener HC, Limmroth V. Lamotrigine reduces migraine aura and migraine attacks in patients with migraine with aura. J Neurol Neurosurg Psychiatry. 2005;76:1730–2.
11. D'Andrea G, Granella F, Cadaldicini N, Manzoni GC. Effectiveness of lamotrigine in the prophylaxis of migraine with aura: an open study. Cephalalgia. 1999;19:64–6.
12. Pascual J, Caminero AB, Mateos V, Roig C, Leira R, García-Moncó C, et al. Preventing disturb-

13. Chen WT, Fuh JL, Lu SR, Wang SJ. Persistent migrainous visual phenomena might be responsive to lamotrigine. Headache. 2001;41:823–5.
14. Reploeg MD, Goebel JA. Migraine-associated dizziness: patient characteristics and management options. Otol Neurotol. 2002;23(3):364–71.
15. Johnson GD. Medical management of migraine-related dizziness and vertigo. Laryngoscope. 1998;108:1–28.
16. Neuhauser H, Lempert T. Vestibular migraine. Neurol Clin. 2009;27(2):379–91.
17. Lempert T, Olesen J, Furman J, et al. Vestibular migraine: diagnostic criteria. J Vestib Res. 2012;22(4):167–72.
18. Neuhauser H, Radtke A, von Brevern M, Lempert T. Zolmitriptan for treatment of migrainous vertigo: a pilot randomized placebo controlled trial. Neurology. 2003;60:882–3.
19. Bikhazi P, Jackson C, Ruckenstein MJ. Efficacy of antimigrainous therapy in the treatment of migraine-associated dizziness. Am J Otol. 1997;18(3):350–4.
20. Prakash S, Shah ND. Migrainous vertigo responsive to intravenous methylprednisolone: case reports. Headache. 2009;49(8):1235–9.
21. Rozen DT. Treatment of prolonged migrainous aura with intravenous furosemide. Neurology. 2000;55:732–3.
22. Haan J, Sluis P, Sluis LH, Ferrari MD. Acetazolamide treatment for migraine aura status. Neurology. 2000;55:1588–9.
23. Ramadan NM. Current trends in migraine prophylaxis. Headache. 2007;47 Suppl 1:S52–7.
24. Maione A. Migraine-related vertigo: diagnostic criteria and prophylactic treatment. Laryngoscope. 2006;116:1782–6.
25. Bisdorff AR. Treatment of migraine related vertigo with lamotrigine an observational study. Bull Soc Sci Med Grand Duche Luxemb. 2004;2:103–8.
26. Cologno D, d'Onofrio F, Castriota O, Petretta V, Casucci G, Russo A, Bussone G. Basilar-type migraine patients responsive to lamotrigine: a 5-year follow-up. Neurol Sci. 2013;34 Suppl 1:S165–6.
27. Celiker A, Bir LS, Ardic̦ N. Effects of valproate on vestibular symptoms and electronystagmographic findings in migraine patients. Clin Neuropharmacol. 2007;30:213–7.
28. Carmona S, Settecase N. Use of topiramate (Topamax) in a subgroup of migraine-vertigo patients with auditory symptoms. Ann N Y Acad Sci. 2005;1039:517–20.
29. Gode S, Celebisoy N, Kirazli T, Akyuz A, Bilgen C, Karapolat H, Sirin H, Gokcay F. Clinical assessment of topiramate therapy in patients with migrainous vertigo. Headache. 2010;50(1):77–84.
30. Lampl C, Bonelli S, Ransmayr G. Efficacy of topiramate in migraine aura prophylaxis: preliminary results of 12 patients. Headache. 2004;44(2):174–6.
31. Brighina F, Palermo A, Aloisio A, Francolini M, Giglia G, Fierro B. Levetiracetam in the prophylaxis

of migraine with aura: a 6-month open-label study. Clin Neuropharmacol. 2006;29(6):338–42.

32. Baier B, Winkenwerder E, Dieterich M. 'Vestibular migraine': effects of prophylactic therapy with various drugs. A retrospective study. J Neurol. 2009;256:436–42.

33. Mikulec AA, Faraji F, Kinsella LJ. Evaluation of the efficacy of caffeine cessation, nortriptyline, and topiramate therapy in vestibular migraine and complex dizziness of unknown etiology. Am J Otolaryngol. 2012;33(1):121–7.

34. Furman JM, Balaban CD, Jacob RG, Marcus DA. Migraine-anxiety related dizziness (MARD): a new disorder? J Neurol Neurosurg Psychiatry. 2005;76:1–8.

35. Baloh RW, Foster CA, Yue Q, Nelson SF. Familial migraine with vertigo and essential tremor. Neurology. 1996;46:458–60.

36. Baker BJ, Curtis A, Trueblood P, Vangsnes E. Vestibular functioning and migraine: comparing those with and without vertigo to a normal population. J Laryngol Otol. 2013;127(12):1169–76.

37. Vitkovic J, Paine M, Rance G. Neuro-otological findings in patients with migraine- and nonmigraine-related dizziness. Audiol Neurootol. 2008;13(2):113–22.

38. Teggi R, Colombo B, Bernasconi L, Bellini C, Comi G, Bussi M. Migrainous vertigo: results of caloric testing and stabilometric findings. Headache. 2009;49(3):435–44.

39. Whitney SL, Wrisley DM, Brown KE, Furman JM. Physical therapy for migraine-related vestibulopathy and vestibular dysfunction with history of migraine. Laryngoscope. 2000;110(9):1528–34.

40. Wrisley DM, Whitney SL, Furman JM. Vestibular rehabilitation outcomes in patients with a history of migraine. Otol Neurotol. 2002;23(4):483–7.

41. Radtke A, von Brevern M, Neuhauser H, Hottenrott T, Lempert T. Vestibular migraine: long-term follow-up of clinical symptoms and vestibulo-cochlear findings. Neurology. 2012;79(15):1607–14.

Ménière's Disease with Concomitant Vestibular Migraine

6

Brian A. Neff and Matthew L. Carlson

6.1 Introduction

The coincidence of Ménière's disease and migraine was first observed by Prosper Ménière in the 1800s. Amazingly, nearly a century passed before renewed interest in this comorbidity resurfaced [1, 2]. Only recently have epidemiological studies looked at their coexistence and clinical presentation overlap. Ménière's disease and vestibular migraine seem to coexist in 28 % of Ménière's disease patients with large clinical overlap in vertigo and associated aural symptom presentation [3]. Although many attempts have been made, there is no objective test or genetic marker to distinguish Ménière's disease from vestibular migraine. Meticulous patient history and audiogram data continue to be the gold standard for the diagnosis of Ménière's disease, vestibular migraine, and Ménière's disease with concomitant vestibular migraine (MDVM). The most distinguishing clinical characteristic for diagnosis of Ménière's disease is the pure-tone average (PTA) and audiometry standards set forth by the 1995 American Academy of Otolaryngology Committee on Hearing and Equilibrium [4]. The most distinguishing features of vestibular migraine are moderate to severe headache and photophobia during vestibular symptoms [3]. Treatment options are currently guided by expert opinion, which can vary. The medical community awaits clinical trials to establish best treatment practices.

6.2 Epidemiology

Epidemiological studies have been very important in the diagnosis and treatment of Ménière's disease and vestibular migraine. Currently, the incidence of Ménière's disease is estimated at 15 cases per 100,000 per year with a prevalence of 218 cases per 100,000 persons or 650,000 current US citizens [5]. Familial Ménière's disease accounts for a minority of Ménière's disease patients, occurring in approximately 7 % of cases, following an autosomal dominant pattern with an estimated 60 % penetrance [6]. Migraine headache and vestibular migraine are much more common than Ménière's disease. Migraine headache prevalence is 15–17 % for women and 6 % for men [7]. Furthermore, migraine headache is seen in 9.7 % of girls and 6 % of boys under 20 years of age [8]. Most importantly for this chapter, the incidence of vestibular migraine in the world population has been estimated at 1–2 % [9]. This is a massive number of vestibular migraine sufferers, which include three to six million US citizens based on current population statistics.

B.A. Neff, MD (✉) • M.L. Carlson, MD
Department of Otolaryngology Head
and Neck Surgery, Mayo Clinic,
200 First St., SW, Rochester, MN 55905, USA
e-mail: neff.brian@mayo.edu;
Carlson.matthew@mayo.edu

S. Wetmore, A. Rubin (eds.), *Vestibular Migraine*,
DOI 10.1007/978-3-319-14550-1_6, © Springer International Publishing Switzerland 2015

The mean age of migraine headache onset is 28 years old while the average age of vertigo onset with vestibular migraine is 49 [10]. A prospective study of 78 patients evaluating the lifetime prevalence of migraine in Ménière's disease compared to an age- and sex-matched control group found that 44 out of 78 (56 %) Ménière's disease patients also had migraine headache compared to 20 out of 78 (25 %) control patients ($p<0.001$) [11]. The prevalence of Ménière's disease in migraine patients has also been studied. A higher than expected proportion of migraine headache patients had Ménière's disease compared to a published prevalence in the general population [2, 12, 13].

6.3   Genetics and Basic Science

Significantly more research has been done for the genetics of sporadic and familial forms of migraine headache than for vestibular migraine. Unfortunately, a vestibular migraine loci or candidate gene has not been isolated. In a similar conundrum, several loci and candidate genes have been proposed in Ménière's disease studies, but a lack of consistent results and reproduction of study findings has hampered significant progress [6]. Cha et al. reported six extensive family pedigrees with migraine, vestibular symptoms, and Ménière's disease showing high degrees of inherited linkage suggesting that at least in these families, there is an underlying genetic determinant. They suggested a genetic basis that links vestibular migraine and Ménière's disease, and it is likely heterogenous and polygenic and confers susceptibility rather than determining disease development [14]. In other words, although purely speculative, Ménière's disease and vestibular migraine may eventually be found to have the same underlying genetic susceptibility with different environmental and epigenetic factors explaining the differences seen along a phenotypic vertigo spectrum.

6.4   Differential Diagnosis

The differential diagnosis of concomitant Ménière's disease and vestibular migraine (MDVM) can be vast when considering pathologies that can cause

Table 6.1 Differential diagnosis of Ménière's disease and vestibular migraine (MDVM)

Ménière's disease (MD) (alone)
Vestibular migraine (VM) (alone)
Basilar migraine
Idiopathic intracranial hypertension
Vertebrobasilar insufficiency (VBI)
Benign recurrent vertigo (BRV)
Benign paroxysmal positional vertigo (BPPV) (vertigo lasting seconds)
Cerebellopontine angle (CPA) tumor
Multiple sclerosis (MS)
Cogan's syndrome
AICA/PICA infarct
Otosyphilis
Episodic ataxia type 2 (EA2) syndrome
Autoimmune inner ear disease (AIED)
Panic attacks
Conversion disorder
Benign paroxysmal vertigo (BPV) of childhood (children)
Juvenile migraine (children)
Enlarged vestibular aqueduct (EVA) (children)
Controversial
Cranial nerve eight vascular compression
Chiari type I malformation
Perilymph fistula

vertigo or headache. However, this section will focus on the more common diagnoses whose patient complaints are both vertigo and headache (Table 6.1).

6.4.1   Basilar Migraine

Patients with basilar migraine make up only a small fraction of all migraine sufferers and there are formal International Headache Society (IHS) criteria for diagnosis [15]. Patients are typically younger women who have an occipital headache that is preceded by less than 1 h of aura. The aura can include typical visual auras, visual field defects, vertigo, dysarthria, diplopia, tinnitus, hearing loss, ataxia, bilateral paresthesias, mental status changes, or bilateral limb weakness. The reason basilar migraine can occasionally be confused with MDVM is that MDVM can include symptoms of migraine headache, vertigo, tinnitus, and, rarely, a transient low-frequency sensorineural hearing loss (SNHL) [16, 17].

6.4.2 Idiopathic Intracranial Hypertension

Idiopathic intracranial hypertension has gone by many previous names such as benign intracranial hypertension and pseudotumor cerebri. It typically presents in women aged 20–40 years with an elevated body mass index (BMI) ≥ 25 kg/m^2. Holocephalic headache without migrainous features and low-tone SNHL and vertigo have been reported, explaining why idiopathic intracranial hypertension is included in the differential for MDVM. Up to 25 % of untreated patients can develop vision loss or blindness. Other symptoms include pulsatile tinnitus, nausea, vomiting, nonspecific dizziness, imbalance, and visual flashes of light (scotomas). Patients do not have focal neurologic deficits or mental status changes. An MRI with a partial or completely empty sella turcica is suggestive of elevated intracranial pressure, but the diagnosis requires that the modified Dandy criteria be met, including: symptoms of increased intracranial pressure, non-focal neurologic exam with the exception of abducens palsy, normal mental status, normal imaging studies (not including empty sella on MRI), lumbar puncture opening pressures of greater than 250 mm H$_2$O without cytological or chemical abnormality, and no other explanation for raised intracranial pressure [18]. Although many physicians rely heavily on the presence or absence of ocular papilledema as a diagnostic screening, it is absent in 5–10 % of confirmed cases [19].

6.4.3 Vertebrobasilar Insufficiency

Vertebrobasilar insufficiency (VBI) is an intracranial posterior circulation transient ischemic attack (TIA), which, if left untreated, can lead to posterior cerebral infarction (anterior inferior cerebellar artery (AICA) or posterior inferior cerebellar artery (PICA) infarct). Most patients are over the age of 60 years and also have atherosclerotic risk factors such as smoking, high cholesterol, and hypertension. Multiple spontaneous bouts of vertigo can occur that usually last less than 20 min but can be longer. Clusters of attacks have been reported. Many times vertigo is brought on by neck extension; however, this is not always necessary. Around 19 % of patients present with vertigo without associated symptoms such as diplopia, visual loss, visual field deficit, dysarthria, dysphagia, mental status changes, or extremity weakness or clumsiness. Finally, headaches occur in 14 % of patients, explaining its inclusion in the differential diagnosis of MDVM. If isolated and repetitive vertigo has occurred for over 6 months without additional symptoms appearing, then VBI is unlikely to be the diagnosis [17, 20]. VBI diagnosis is usually confirmed with MRI/MRA or CT angiogram.

6.4.4 Benign Recurrent Vertigo

Benign recurrent vertigo (BRV) is a diagnosis given to patients with recurrent spontaneous vertigo that demonstrates overlapping features with vestibular migraine, Ménière's disease, or MDVM; however BRV patients do not meet formal diagnostic criteria for any of these conditions. This is usually due to a lack of documented audiometric hearing loss or consistent timing between vertigo spells and migrainous symptoms. BRV has suffered from a lack of consistent nomenclature (chronic vestibulopathy, recurrent vestibulopathy, vestibular Ménière's disease) and diagnostic validity. However, the stricter the vestibular migraine and Ménière's disease criteria get, the more patients will default into this category. A few studies have shown that most of these patient's symptoms will spontaneously resolve and do not evolve into Ménière's disease [21, 22]. Similarly, most of these patients have migraine symptoms, such as photophobia, or strong family histories of migraine and, thus, from a practical clinical standpoint should be treated similar to vestibular migraine [14].

6.5 Hypotheses Concerning Comorbidity

6.5.1 Endolymphatic Hydrops

In 1938, Hallpike and Cairns performed an autopsy study and established the histopathologic description of endolymphatic hydrops (EH) in temporal bones of patients with Ménière's disease [23]. In a more recent meta-analysis, 541 temporal bone specimens with EH were analyzed and 276 (51 %) of these were found to have clinical Ménière's disease by varying criteria. When applying the more strict diagnostic criteria set forth by the 1995 American Academy of Otolaryngology (AAO) Committee on Hearing and Equilibrium Ménière's disease criteria, 98.8 % (163/165) of Ménière's disease patients had EH, otherwise defined as certain Ménière's disease. Of the 276 patients diagnosed with Ménière's disease by varying criteria, 111 (40 %) of them did not meet the 1995 AAO criteria. Of these, 106/111 (95 %) had EH despite not having Ménière's disease. The authors postulated that many of the EH patients not meeting the 1995 AAO Ménière's disease criteria had fluctuating or progressive hearing loss without vertigo or had vertigo without documented hearing loss [4, 24]. A major problem with the authors' assertion is that the clinical descriptions of vertigo from Ménière's disease and vestibular migraine are often indistinguishable. None of the patients in the temporal bone meta-analysis were evaluated with vestibular migraine clinical criteria, and while not all of these patients had vestibular migraine, epidemiology statistics would suggest that at least some of them did. Consequently, it is possible that some percentage of vestibular migraine patients have EH. Temporal bone studies utilizing vestibular migraine diagnostic criteria are needed.

If vestibular migraine patients demonstrate EH, it is unknown if the presence or absence of EH is a predictor of later development of Ménière's disease in addition to the vestibular migraine. Many vestibular migraine patients have isolated otologic symptoms such as tinnitus or aural fullness, which do not seem to predict Ménière's disease development. Although controversial, a few have mild fluctuating SNHL while maintaining good speech discrimination scores. Could EH be a possible explanation for this? A natural question follows: does EH develop from repetitive ischemic episodes from vestibular migraine, and is Ménière's disease just a more advanced disease presentation given the greater degree of hearing loss, the often permanent hearing loss, and the frequent vestibular hypofunction? Conversely, do vestibular migraine and EH occur independently due to another mechanism such as a channelopathy that leads to Ménière's disease? Why do many vestibular migraine patients who may or may not have EH not develop Ménière's disease? These and many other unproven hypotheses and unanswered questions will hopefully be answered or refuted with future research.

6.5.2 Ischemia

Transient changes in inner ear perfusion could cause vertigo in migraine patients, and repetitive vascular ischemia could lead to permanent cochleovestibular damage and symptoms seen in Ménière's disease [11, 14]. It is unknown if the proposed decline in perfusion is from vasospasm of cochlear arteries (intralabyrinthine artery) or arterioles in a manner similar to the rare phenomenon of retinal artery vasospasm and retinal migraine [25]. Another hypothesis is that EH can create increased resistance to blood flow and change autoregulation of microvasculature within the cochlea and labyrinth [26].

Foster et al. present logical, but as yet, unproven hypotheses for the physiology of Ménière's disease and its interrelatedness to migraine. They postulated that preexisting EH is necessary but not sufficient to cause Ménière's disease; however, they did not explain why EH develops. The patients must also have a heightened risk for intracerebral and intra-aural ischemia caused by such diseases as migraine, otosyphilis, and neuroborreliosis. Finally, the symptoms seen in Ménière's disease are from inner ear tissues that are differentially sensitive to inner ear ischemia, particularly the apical stria vascularis in the cochlea. They hypothesized that any disease process that can cause decreased intracerebral arterial pressure, increased venous outflow resistance, or chronically raised intracerebral CSF pressure can provide heightened ischemia risk. They state that EH is not caused by ischemia and vascular risk factors do not result from EH, i.e., EH and vascular risk factors are related by chance [24]. Unfortunately, this is not consistent with epidemiologic data where migraine and Ménière's disease are not chance co-occurrences.

6.5.3   Channelopathy

Since there is evidence that episodic ataxia syndromes and hemiplegic migraine result from channelopathies, many authors have recently hypothesized that Ménière's disease and vestibular migraine may result from a similar pathogenesis. Ménière's disease and vestibular migraine might be caused by a defective ion channel selectively expressed in neuronal and inner ear tissues. This would cause cortical spreading depression in migraine and toxic increases of perilymphatic potassium in the inner ear in Ménière's disease [11]. Further supporting this hypothesis is the observation that most potassium and calcium channelopathies produce adult-onset, paroxysmal symptoms, which are patterns consistent with vestibular migraine and Ménière's disease [27]. However, actual genetic, histologic, or pathophysiologic evidence for this hypothesis is currently lacking.

6.5.4   Central Mechanisms of Migraine Dizziness and Sterile Inflammation of the Inner Ear

Central mechanisms of vertigo play a major role in vestibular migraine pathophysiology. The vestibular nuclei receive serotonin-mediated input from the dorsal raphe nucleus and noradrenergic input from the locus ceruleus, which are both areas of the brain heavily involved in migraine physiology and, possibly, vertigo generation [28]. The understanding of interconnections between different central migraine and pain pathways and central vestibular circuits is increasingly expanding and complex. These central migraine and vestibular pathways may also interact with the peripheral end organ, the inner ear. In addition to triggering spreading cortical depression, the trigeminovascular system is definitively implicated

in the development of migraine pain and has been found to innervate the vasculature of the inner ear [29]. The trigeminovascular reflex has been shown to cause sterile inflammation of the dura mater and the perivascular tissue of the basilar and anterior inferior cerebellar artery in animal models. Recent studies have shown a similar plasma/protein extravasation from the spiral modiolar artery and its arterioles. Koo et al. have shown neurogenic plasma extravasation by activation of the trigeminovascular reflex into the apical spiral ganglion, the modiolus, and the inner ear segments of the vestibular nerves in mice. Similarly, trigeminal sensory afferent fibers are found in very high density within the stria vascularis and, when stimulated, release neuropeptides such as calcitonin gene-related peptide, substance P, and neurokinin A. These neuropeptides induce a vasodilatory response and protein extravasation into the stria vascularis and endolymph [30]. Additionally, neuropeptide release has an excitatory effect on the baseline neural activity of the inner ear [13, 31]. Although not conclusive, this sterile inner ear inflammation might be partly regulated by the main serotonin receptor targets of the triptans (5-HT 1A, 1B, 1D, 1F) which have been documented in the spiral ganglion and vestibular ganglion cells [29]. Koo et al. also hypothesized that this sterile inflammation may cause an osmotic load that could interfere with the potassium recycling mechanism of the inner ear. They did not study the potential ischemic changes, loss of hair cells or stria cells, or development of possible EH after repetitive sterile inflammatory insults [30]. While yet unproven, this hypothesis is very attractive as a potential explanation of auditory symptoms with vestibular migraine and possibly the development of EH or Ménière's disease in the human patient.

6.6   Overlap in Clinical Presentation and Testing

A primary difficulty in diagnosing and categorizing Ménière's disease and vestibular migraine is that some physicians have not adopted the Bárány classification of vestibular symptoms that are at the core of Ménière's disease and vestibular migraine definition [32]. Furthermore, there is yet no universal agreement as to which vertigo descriptions should be included in "typical" Ménière's disease and vestibular migraine dizziness attacks. An example of such, Sargent used the Bárány definition of internal vertigo which is described as a "sense of self-motion when no motion is occurring, or the sensation of distorted self-motion during an otherwise normal head movement" when describing Ménière's disease vertigo [8]. This definition did not include external vertigo, which is "a false sensation that the visual surround is spinning or flowing" which most physicians would also include [32]. Another problem with the definitions when applied to Ménière's disease and vestibular migraine is that certain descriptions of internal or external vertigo do not likely belong in Ménière's disease or vestibular migraine disease classification. An example of such includes this description of internal vertigo: "there is a spinning inside of my head; or it feels as if my brain is turning within my skull." This sensation of internal vertigo is more likely described with conversion disorder and does not fall into most clinician's definition of Ménière's disease or vestibular migraine-like vertigo. Lastly, physicians have the problem that the patient may not be able to reliably discriminate these subtleties and relay them accurately. It is the author's experience that many cannot.

Increasing recognition of vestibular migraine criteria such as the Neuhauser criteria or the most recent Bárány and IHS society definition can only help to better categorize these patients for prognosis and treatment trials [33, 34]. However, there are some issues with these criteria when it comes to treating everyday Ménière's disease, vestibular migraine, and MDVM patients. The regular temporal pattern of migraine headache and vestibular symptoms is absent in 30–50 % of reported vestibular migraine patients, and up to 30 % of patients eventually diagnosed with vestibular migraine will initially present without headache [12, 35]. Alternatively, vestibular migraine criteria have increasingly demanded this temporal relationship with the exclusion of greater numbers of patients. As mentioned, this will likely be helpful in studying the natural course of vestibular migraine and treatment effects by ensuring a greater purity in vestibular migraine patient inclusion. However, in the clinical arena, this has left an increasing number of patients without a diagnosis or at least an attempt at empirical treatment for vestibular migraine. Hopefully, the increasing exclusion of these patients will lead to the discovery of a new diagnostic phenotype rather than including them in "waste basket" diagnoses such as BRV or shifting them to other vertigo diagnoses that equally do not fit such as Ménière's disease or BPPV.

Another major clinical challenge is that there is currently no history, physical exam, vestibular test, or imaging finding that is pathognomonic for Ménière's disease alone, vestibular migraine alone, or MDVM [12]. This may be from a limitation in the current classification systems and limitations in current testing capabilities and technology, or it may be that these two entities are not distinguishable and are slightly different phenotypic presentations of an underlying unifying pathophysiology. More research is necessary to clarify the definitions in the future. Clearly certain historical points build evidentiary support for vestibular migraine, Ménière's disease, or MDVM, but significant exceptions always exist for the clinician. For example, classic Ménière's disease symptoms of subjective fluctuating or progressive hearing loss, tinnitus, and aural fullness occur in vestibular migraine patients 36, 55, and 51 % of the time, respectively. Conversely, vestibular migraine symptoms of headache, photophobia episodes, and aura occur in 81, 40, and 22 % of Ménière's disease sufferers who do not meet formal vestibular migraine criteria [3]. As a common practice, vestibular testing is frequently used to rule Ménière's disease "in or out," but this is not really possible since many Ménière's disease patients have normal vestibular testing results, especially early in the disease process. Additionally, vestibular migraine patients have abnormalities in VNG, rotary chair, VEMP, and ECoG in up to 15–35 % of patients [3, 12, 14, 36, 37]. Newer tests such as ocular VEMP (oVEMP) and intratympanic gadolinium-enhanced MRI scans hold some promise for help in distinguishing vestibular migraine and Ménière's disease. However, early reports are also showing overlaps in abnormalities in Ménière's disease and vestibular migraine patients. Zuniga et al. were unable to find any cVEMP or oVEMP test that could distinguish between Ménière's disease and vestibular migraine [38]. Additionally, 19 consecutive definite and probable vestibular migraine patients without Ménière's disease or hearing loss were scanned with intratympanic gadolinium-enhanced MRI technique, and 4 (19 %) were found to have endolymphatic hydrops [39]. Currently, the 1995 AAO Ménière's disease guidelines should be used to diagnose Ménière's disease, and the Bárány society criteria should be used for vestibular migraine [4, 32]. If the patient meets the criteria for both, then the diagnosis of MDVM should be made. Objective SNHL criteria for low-tone PTA per the 1995 AAO Ménière's disease guidelines are the most specific criteria for Ménière's disease diagnosis. Future Ménière's disease criterion revisions might consider adding speech discrimination score requirements to the audiologic requirements. Finally, a history of moderate or severe headache and photophobia during vertigo spells was the most specific diagnostic history point for vestibular migraine diagnosis [3].

6.7 Treatment

6.7.1 Comorbid Ménière's Disease and Vestibular Migraine

Currently, there are no published outcome studies evaluating the best practice treatment approaches for MDVM. Generally speaking, there are two reasonable approaches to consider. The authors' preferred approach is to treat the vestibular migraine component first with dietary modification and prophylactic migraine medications (Fig. 6.1). There are several reasons supporting this strategy. First, treatment risk is really limited to medication side effects, and these are nearly always self-limited with reduction or termination of medical therapy (Table 6.2). Vestibular migraine medical treatment does not expose patients to the permanent risks of hearing loss

and worsened disequilibrium that are associated with intratympanic injection and surgical Ménière's disease therapies. Second, some migraine prophylactics may have beneficial treatment effects for Ménière's disease, such as calcium channel blockers [40]. Lastly, many of these patients have comorbid chronic subjective dizziness and health anxiety issues that make them less than ideal candidates for procedural or surgical interventions until these issues are resolved.

The second reasonable treatment strategy is to first treat Ménière's disease or vestibular migraine based on the predominance of symptom support for either diagnoses. In cases where Ménière's disease is felt to be playing a primary role in vertigo persistence, the authors favor medical therapy with diuretics and salt-restricted diet as a first-line therapy. If this conservative approach fails, then the authors utilize non-ablative Ménière's disease treatments as second-line therapies. Non-ablative therapies include intratympanic steroid injections, Meniett device use, or endolymphatic sac surgery. Many of these patients have bilateral ear symptomology and bilateral vestibular test abnormalities and may be at higher risk to develop contralateral Ménière's disease even if they are currently presenting with unilateral disease complaints [41]. The last point is a very important concern that should at least be considered during treatment planning. Unfortunately, clear-cut evidence of efficacy has not been identified for non-ablative therapies. Cochrane reviews (systematic meta-analysis) have been performed for Ménière's disease medical therapies and, to date, have not found any support for the effectiveness of diuretic, low-sodium diet, or betahistine [42, 43]. The fact that effectiveness was not demonstrated does not mean that there is clear evidence that these medical therapies do not work; consequently, diuretic, low-sodium diet, and betahistine continue to be used for Ménière's disease treatment by most neurotologists. A Cochrane review of intratympanic steroids in January 2011 found only one small prospective, randomized, blinded, placebo-controlled trial that had an acceptable risk of bias. In this study, 22 patients were randomized and the treatment group received 5 injections of

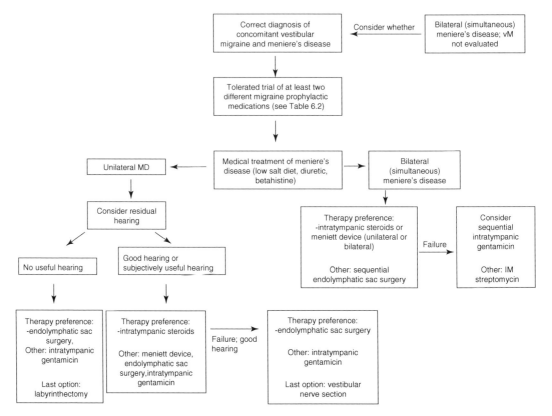

Fig. 6.1 Management algorithm for concomitant Ménière's disease and vestibular migraine (MDVM). Key: *IM* intramuscular, *VM* vestibular migraine, *MD* Ménière's disease

4 mg/ml dexamethasone in 5 days (once per day). The authors demonstrated a significant reduction in vertigo at 24 months in the treatment group as measured by AAO-HNS functional level, vertigo class (AAO-HNS definition), Dizziness Handicap Inventory (DHI) score, and subjective vertigo improvement [44, 45]. Endolymphatic sac shunting or decompression can also be done for non-ablative Ménière's disease vertigo treatment. The effectiveness of this treatment is highly controversial; however, it is still a widely accepted practice within the neurotology community [46]. MDVM patients should be cautioned about the potential for lower success rates since patients with Ménière's disease alone may do much better with endolymphatic sac surgery than those with MDVM in regard to postoperative QOL measures [8].

With either approach, a few MDVM patients will be treatment resistant to initial therapies. It should be noted that not tolerating a vestibular migraine prophylactic medication is not a failed medication trial and every effort should be made to identify a medication class that is tolerable to the patient. In cases where MDVM patients continue to have spontaneous vertigo of >20 min duration and have failed at least two different classes of migraine prophylactic medications (Table 6.2) and non-ablative Ménière's disease treatments, then the author favors intratympanic gentamicin given via a titration method. This approach often leads to vertigo control without completely ablating the vestibular system. This may be important if the contralateral ear develops Ménière's disease in the future. Titrated intratympanic gentamicin can be used after failed medical and non-ablative treatments in the second ear due to the residual, yet reduced, vestibular function that was maintained in the initial ear after previous intratympanic gentamicin. The patient does need to be

Table 6.2 Prophylactic medications for the treatment of vestibular migraine with or without concomitant Ménière's disease

Medication	Drug class	Starting dose	Goal dose	Maximum dose	Titration	Common side effects
Topiramate (Topamax)	Anticonvulsant	25 mg QD	50 mg BID	200 mg BID	Increase by 25 mg every 7 days	Word finding difficulty, trouble concentrating, mental fogginess, weight loss, tingling in extremities
Venlafaxine XR (Effexor XR)	Serotonin-norepinephrine reuptake inhibitor (SNRI)	37.5 mg QD	75–150 mg QD	225 mg QD	Increase by 37.5 mg every 14 days	Drug withdrawal, headache exacerbation, increased blood pressure, perioral or extremity tingling, vivid dreams, sexual dysfunction, suicidal ideation
Gabapentin (Neurontin)	Anticonvulsant	300 mg QD	600 mg TID	1,200 mg TID	Increase by 300 mg per day every 7 days	Drowsiness, dizziness, unsteadiness, weight gain, fatigue, extremity fluid retention, blurred vision
Nortriptyline (Pamelor)	Tricyclic antidepressant	10 mg QHS	50–70 mg QHS	150 mg QHS	Increase by 10 mg every 7 days	Dry mouth, constipation, weight gain, fatigue, somnolence
Verapamil (Verelan)	Calcium channel blocker	120 mg QD	240 mg QD	240 mg BID; caution arrhythmia	Increase by 60 mg every 7 days	Constipation, palpitations, peripheral edema, hypotension, fatigue
Metoprolol (Toprol XL)	Beta blocker	25 mg QD	100 mg QD	400 mg QD	Increase by 25 mg every 7 days	Fatigue, bradycardia, cold hands and feet, hypotension, depression, weight gain, decreased libido, impotence, vivid dreams, difficulty breathing, constipation/diarrhea, upset stomach Caution: patients with CHF, COPD, asthma, diabetes

counseled about the risk of imbalance and oscillopsia that can occur in a minority of patients after bilateral partial vestibular ablation. Although very effective for vertigo control, vestibular nerve section and labyrinthectomy both lead to complete vestibular ablation in the initially treated ear and cannot be done in both ears without resulting in disabling oscillopsia. Although not definitively proven, the authors' anecdotal experience is that this MDVM group has a much higher rate of initial and eventual bilateral Ménière's disease development. Intramuscular streptomycin has been successfully used in past bilateral Ménière's disease case series; however, streptomycin is not easily available or familiar to most contemporary physicians. The authors favor sequential (right ear and then 6 weeks later left ear or vice versa) bilateral intratympanic gentamicin injections followed by vestibular rehabilitation for patients with treatment-resistant MDVM whether it be bilateral simultaneous or bilateral sequential ear presentation. The ear to be injected first in cases of bilateral simultaneous presentation is primarily decided by which ear has the predominant symptoms while factoring in which ear has the worst hearing and greatest vestibular hypofunction. Simultaneous (both ears at the same visit) intratympanic gentamicin in bilateral Ménière's disease or MDVM cases has not been tried, to date, by the authors or reported in the literature.

6.7.2 Concern over Bilateral Ménière's Disease

Not much is known about why bilateral Ménière's disease occurs and who is at risk. Relevant to this chapter is, are MDVM patients potentially at more risk to develop bilateral Ménière's disease? Bilateral Ménière's disease rarely presents with bilateral simultaneous disease; rather, most patients experience sequential involvement of both ears over time. There is disagreement in the literature with some researchers claiming that most cases of bilateral Ménière's disease develop in the second ear within 2–5 years. Others believe that there is a steady increase in the incidence over one's entire lifetime [47]. A large Japanese

study of 1,368 Ménière's disease cases found that the incidence of bilateral Ménière's disease increased from 9.2 to 16.2 % in over 30 years [48]. This factor of time, differing patient populations and selection bias, and loose application of Ménière's disease and vestibular migraine diagnostic criteria have likely led to the large variation of reported incidence (5–33 %) of bilateral Ménière's disease [49, 50]. Currently, we do not firmly know if MDVM or even Ménière's disease without vestibular migraine (with migraine features) has an increased incidence of bilateral Ménière's disease. The authors' paper did not find a higher incidence of bilateral Ménière's disease in MDVM compared to Ménière's disease alone. However, the follow-up time for these patients was primarily under 5 years.

There are a few circumstantial pieces of evidence that probably justify concern for bilateral Ménière's disease development in MDVM patients. Clemmens et al. found that bilateral Ménière's disease patients had a statistically higher rate of migraine headache and family history of Ménière's disease [41]. Our study of MDVM patients found that a significantly higher percentage of MDVM patients had subjective bilateral complaints of hearing loss despite not meeting bilateral Ménière's disease audiometric criteria at 5 years or less [3]. We also saw that MDVM patients had a higher incidence of a family history of vertigo, which according to Clemmens et al. may make them at higher risk for bilateral Ménière's disease development. Moreover, the Japanese study showing an increase of bilateral Ménière's disease incidence over time is concerning since the average onset of MDVM and vestibular migraine is in the early 40s compared with Ménière's disease alone whose average onset was in the 50s [3]. The earlier the onset, the longer the MDVM patient may have to develop bilateral Ménière's disease in the future. Lastly, there have been several studies looking at VEMP tuning curves and thresholds in unilateral Ménière's disease patients to see if bilateral abnormalities can be detected in the asymptomatic ear. One showed that 27 % of contralateral asymptomatic ears had abnormalities consistent with EH. However, the long-term longitudinal studies to assess the predictive value of these tests for the development of clinical bilateral Ménière's disease are still lacking [47, 51]. Although not definitively proven, the authors treat the unilateral MDVM patient and the isolated Ménière's disease patient with some migrainous features with more caution for risk of developing bilateral Ménière's disease in their lifetime. As previously pointed out, migraine prophylactic medications and non-ablative therapies should be exhausted prior to considering ablative Ménière's disease treatment options in this patient population.

Concern over bilateral Ménière's disease is important to both patients and clinicians. From a treatment standpoint, bilateral Ménière's disease limits treatment options because few physicians will offer bilateral complete vestibular ablative procedures, such as labyrinthectomy or vestibular nerve section, due to the resultant disabling oscillopsia. Additionally, bilateral severe hearing loss has to be taken into account, and some of these patients will need cochlear implantation for hearing rehabilitation. Cochlear implantation prohibits transtympanic injections for Ménière's disease treatment due to the electrode blocking access to the round window membrane. Surgical planning can also become more complex in patients who need cochlear implant surgery combined with vertigo control surgery, such as endolymphatic sac surgery [52]. Although simultaneous labyrinthectomy and cochlear implantation has been used successfully in unilateral Ménière's disease patients, the authors prefer cochlear implantation combined with non-ablative endolymphatic sac surgery in this patient population (MDVM) at higher risk for bilateral Ménière's disease [53]. This approach can be used for both ears and may obviate the need for labyrinthectomy in one or both ears; and consequently, labyrinthectomy can hopefully be avoided bilaterally.

6.8 Summary

Ménière's disease and vestibular migraine are comorbid in up to 25 % of patients. History and physical examination are currently the gold standard for distinguishing which of these two diagnoses is correct or if both are contributing to patient morbidity. To date, vestibular testing and imaging cannot reliably distinguish Ménière's disease and vestibular migraine. Management of Ménière's disease with concomitant vestibular migraine often requires prophylactic migraine medication management combined with non-ablative Ménière's disease treatments. Ablative Ménière's disease treatments should be utilized as a last resort, in severely symptomatic patients failing initial conservative treatments. Future clinical studies are needed to establish the most effective treatment protocols for comorbid Ménière's disease and vestibular migraine.

References

1. Atkinson M. Migraine and Ménière's disease. Arch Otolaryngol. 1962;75:220–5.
2. Kayan A, Hood JD. Neuro-otological manifestations of migraine. Brain. 1984;107:1123–42.
3. Neff BA, Staab JP, Carlson ML, et al. Auditory and vestibular symptoms and chronic subjective dizziness in patients with Ménière's disease, vestibular migraine, and Ménière's disease with concomitant vestibular migraine. Otol Neurotol. 2012;33:1235–44.
4. Committee on hearing and equilibrium guidelines for the diagnosis and evaluation of therapy in Ménière's disease. Otolaryngol Head Neck Surg. 1995;113:181–5.
5. Wladislavosky-Waserman P, Facer GW, Mokri B, et al. Ménière's disease: a 30-year epidemiologic & clinical study in Rochester, MN, 1951-80. Laryngoscope. 1984;94(8):1098–102.
6. Vrbec JT. Genetic investigations of Ménière's disease. Otolaryngol Clin North Am. 2010;43(5):1121–32.
7. Lipton RB, Scher AI, Kolodner K, et al. Migraine in the United States: epidemiology and patterns of healthcare use. Neurology. 2002;58(6):885–94.
8. Sargent EW. The challenge of vestibular migraine. Curr Opin Otolaryngol Head Neck Surg. 2013;21:473–9.
9. von Brevern M, Neuhauser H. Epidemiological evidence for a link between vertigo and migraine. J Vestib Res. 2011;21:299–304.
10. Eggers SDZ, Staab JP, Neff BA, et al. Investigation of the coherence of definite and probable vestibular migraine as distinct clinical entities. Otol Neurotol. 2011;32:1144–51.
11. Radtke A, Lempert T, Gresty MA, et al. Migraine and Ménière's disease, is there a link? Neurology. 2002; 59:1700–4.
12. Shepard NT. Differentiation of Ménière's disease and migraine-associated dizziness: a review. J Am Acad Audiol. 2006;17:69–80.

13. Ibekwe TS, Fasunla JA, Ibekwe PU, et al. Migraine and Ménière's disease: two different phenomena with frequently observed concomitant occurrences. J Natl Med Assoc. 2008;100(3):334–8.
14. Cha YH, Kane MJ, Baloh RW. Familial clustering of migraine, episodic vertigo, and Ménière's disease. Otol Neurotol. 2008;29(1):93–6.
15. International Headache Society Classification Sub-committee. International classification of headache disorders. 2nd ed. Cephalalgia. 2004;24 Suppl 1:1–160.
16. Olsson JE. Neurotologic findings in basilar migraine. Laryngoscope. 1991;101(1 Pt 2 Suppl 52):1–41.
17. Karatas M. Vascular vertigo: epidemiology and clinical syndromes. Neurologist. 2011;17:1–10.
18. Friedman DI, Jacobson DM. Diagnostic criteria for idiopathic intracranial hypertension. Neurology. 2002;59:1492–5.
19. Peng KP, Fuh JL, Wang SJ. High-pressure headaches: idiopathic intracranial hypertension and its mimics. Nat Rev Neurol. 2012;8(12):700–12.
20. Ishiyama G, Ishiyama A. Vertebrobasilar infarcts and ischemia. Otolaryngol Clin North Am. 2011;44: 415–35.
21. Lee HK, Ahn SK, Jeon SY, et al. Clinical characteristics and natural course of recurrent vestibulopathy: a long-term follow-up study. Laryngoscope. 2012; 122(4):883–6.
22. Cha YH, Lee H, Santell LS, et al. Association of benign recurrent vertigo and migraine in 208 patients. Cephalalgia. 2009;29(5):550–7.
23. Hallpike C, Cairns H. Observations on the pathology of Ménière's syndrome. J Laryngol Otol. 1938;53: 625–54.
24. Foster CA, Breeze RE. Endolymphatic hydrops in Ménière's disease: cause, consequence, or epiphenomenon. Otol Neurotol. 2013;34:1210–4.
25. Lee H, Lopez I, Ishiyami A, et al. Can migraine damage the inner ear? Arch Neurol. 2000;57:1631–4.
26. Kimura R. Experimental endolymphatic hydrops. In: Harris JP, editor. Ménière's disease. The Hague: Kugler publications; 1999. p. 115–24.
27. Gates P. Hypothesis: could Ménière's disease be a channelopathy? Intern Med J. 2005;35:488–9.
28. Furman JM, Marcus DA, Balaban CD. Migrainous vertigo: development of a pathogenetic model and structured diagnostic interview. Curr Opin Neurol. 2003;16:5–13.
29. Furman JM, Marcus DA, Balaban CD. Vestibular migraine: clinical aspects and pathophysiology. Lancet Neurol. 2013;12:706–15.
30. Koo KW, Balaban CD. Serotonin-induced plasma extravasation in the murine inner ear: possible mechanism of migraine-associated inner ear dysfunction. Cephalalgia. 2006;26:1310–9.
31. Cutrer FM, Baloh RW. Migraine-associated dizziness. Headache. 1992;32(6):300–4.
32. Bisdorff A, Von Brevern M, Lempert T, et al. Classification of vestibular symptoms: towards an international classification of vestibular disorders. J Vestib Res. 2009;19:1–13.
33. Neuhauser H, Lempert T. Vestibular migraine. Neurol Clin. 2009;27:379–91.
34. Lempert T, Olesen J, Furman J, et al. Vestibular migraine: diagnostic criteria. J Vestib Res. 2012;22: 167–72.
35. Strupp M, Versino M, Brandt T. Vestibular migraine. Handb Clin Neurol. 2010;97:755–71.
36. Wuyts FL, Van de Heyning PH, Van Spaendonck MP, et al. A review of electrocochleography: instrumentation settings and meta-analysis of criteria for diagnosis of endolymphatic hydrops. Acta Otolaryngol Suppl. 1997;526:14–20.
37. Johnson GD. Medical management of migraine-related dizziness and vertigo. Laryngoscope. 1998; 108(1 Pt 2):1–28.
38. Zuniga MG, Janky KL, Schubert MC, et al. Can vestibular-evoked myogenic potentials help differentiate Ménière's disease from vestibular migraine. Otolaryngol Head Neck Surg. 2012;145(5): 788–96.
39. Gurkov R, Katner C, Strupp M, et al. Endolymphatic hydrops in patients with vestibular migraine and auditory symptoms. Eur Arch Otorhinolaryngol. 2014; 271(10):2661–7.
40. Lassen LF, Hirsch BE, Kamerer DB. Use of nimodipine in the medical treatment of Ménière's disease: clinical experience. Am J Otol. 1996;17:577–80.
41. Clemmens C, Ruckenstein M. Characteristics of patients with unilateral and bilateral Ménière's disease. Otol Neurotol. 2012;33(7):1266–9.
42. Burgess A, Kundu S. Diuretics for Ménière's disease or syndrome (review). Cochrane Database Syst Rev. 2006 (3):CD003599. Updated 2010, Issue 4.
43. James A, Burton MJ. Betahistine for Ménière's disease or syndrome (review). Cochrane Database Syst Rev. 2001 (1):CD001873. Updated 2011, Issue 3.
44. Phillips JS, Westerberg B. Intratympanic steroids for Ménière's disease or syndrome. Cochrane Database Syst Rev. 2011 (7):CD008514.
45. Garduno-Anaya MA, Couthino De Toledo H, Hinojosa GR, Pane PC, Rios Castenada LC. Dexamethasone inner ear perfusion by intratympanic injection in unilateral Ménière's disease: a two-year prospective, placebo-controlled, double-blind, randomized trial. Otolaryngol Head Neck Surg. 2005; 133(2):285–94.
46. Kim HH, Wiet RJ, Battista RA. Trends in the management of Ménière's disease: results of a survey. Otolaryngol Head Neck Surg. 2005;132(5):72–6.
47. Nabi S, Parnes LS. Bilateral Ménière's disease. Curr Opin Otolaryngol Head Neck Surg. 2009;17:356–62.
48. Shojaku H, Wantanabe Y, Yagi T, et al. Changes in the characteristics of definite Ménière's disease over time in Japan: a long-term survey by the Peripheral Vestibular Disorder Research Committee of Japan. Acta Otolaryngol. 2009;129:155–60.

49. Perez R, Chen JM, Nedzelski JM. The status of the contralateral ear in established unilateral Ménière's disease. Laryngoscope. 2004;114:1373–6.

50. Chaves AG, Boari L, Lei Munhoz MS. The outcome of patients with Ménière's disease. Braz J Otorhinolaryngol. 2007;73:346–50.

51. Lin MY, Timmer FC, Oriel BS, et al. Vestibular evoked myogenic potentials (VEMP) can detect asymptomatic saccular hydrops. Laryngoscope. 2006;116:987–92.

52. Holden LK, Neely JG, Gotter BD, et al. Sequential bilateral cochlear implantation in a patient with bilateral Ménière's disease. J Am Acad Audiol. 2012; 23(4):256–68.

53. Hansen MR, Gantz BJ, Dunn C. Outcomes after cochlear implantation for patients with single-sided deafness, including those with recalcitrant Ménière's disease. Otol Neurotol. 2013;34(9):1681–7.

Printed in the United States
By Bookmasters